**Understanding
Intracardiac
EGMs and ECGs**

To Howard and Sumiko Kusumoto

Understanding Intracardiac EGMs and ECGs

Fred Kusumoto, MD

Associate Professor of Medicine
Mayo School of Medicine
Director of Pacing and Electrophysiology
Division of Cardiovascular Diseases
Mayo Clinic
Jacksonville, FL, USA

WILEY-BLACKWELL

A John Wiley & Sons, Ltd., Publication

This edition first published 2010 © 2010 Fred Kusumoto

Blackwell Publishing was acquired by John Wiley & Sons in February 2007. Blackwell's publishing program has been merged with Wiley's global Scientific, Technical and Medical business to form Wiley-Blackwell.

Registered office: John Wiley & Sons Ltd, The Atrium, Southern Gate, Chichester, West Sussex, PO19 8SQ, UK

Editorial offices: 9600 Garsington Road, Oxford, OX4 2DQ, UK
The Atrium, Southern Gate, Chichester, West Sussex, PO19 8SQ, UK
111 River Street, Hoboken, NJ 07030-5774, USA

For details of our global editorial offices, for customer services and for information about how to apply for permission to reuse the copyright material in this book please see our website at www.wiley.com/wiley-blackwell

Library of Congress Cataloging-in-Publication Data
Kusumoto, Fred.
    Understanding intracardiac EGMs and ECG's / by Fred Kusumoto.
       p.   ;   cm.
    Includes index.
    ISBN 978-1-4051-8410-6
    1. Electrocardiography.   2. Heart–Electric properties.   I. Title.
    [DNLM: 1. Electrophysiologic Techniques, Cardiac–methods.   2. Electrocardiography–methods.
WG 141.5.F9 K97u 2009]
    RC683.5.E5K87 2009
    616.1'207547–dc22

                                                                                              2009013387

ISBN: 9781405184106

A catalogue record for this book is available from the British Library.

Set in 9.5/12pt Palatino by Graphicraft Limited, Hong Kong
Printed and bound in Malaysia

1   2010

Contents

Preface, vii

Part 1 Electrophysiology Concepts

1 Procedural issues for electrophysiologic studies: vascular access, cardiac chamber access, and catheters, 3

2 Fluoroscopic anatomy and electrophysiologic recording in the heart, 15

3 Programmed stimulation, 29

4 Bradycardia, 51

5 Supraventricular tachycardia, 60

6 Wide complex tachycardia, 86

7 New technology, 94

8 Power sources for ablation, 99

Part 2 Specific Arrhythmias

9 Accessory pathways, 107

10 AV node reentry, 132

11 Focal atrial tachycardia, 148

12 Atrial flutter, 161

13 Atrial fibrillation, 182

14 Ventricular tachycardia, 189

15 Implantable cardiac devices: ECGs and electrograms, 211

Index, 220

Preface

Electrophysiology has evolved from a field populated by the "nerds of medicine" to an essential mainstream specialty area within cardiology. Still, much of electrophysiology remains clouded in mystery. Although the electrocardiogram (ECG) is accepted as a standard clinical tool, electrograms (EGMs) recorded during electrophysiology studies are considered complex and confusing. However, since electrograms and the ECG both measure the same thing – electrical activity of the heart – they provide synergistic information. In fact the specialized electrode catheters that are used to acquire intracardiac electrograms can simply be thought of as ECG leads that are within the heart rather than on the skin surface. It is with this relationship in mind that this book attempts to use electrograms and the ECG to discuss rhythm disorders of the heart and provide the newcomer with an introductory guide to electrophysiology studies and the interpretation of electrograms.

The book is divided into two broad sections. In the first section, the basics of electrophysiology testing are reviewed, along with the diagnostic evaluation of general types of arrhythmias such as bradycardia, supraventricular tachycardia, and wide complex tachycardia. Although the chapter discussing the electrophysiological evaluation of supraventricular tachycardia may appear daunting, once the basic tenets are understood, electrophysiology techniques provide a wonderful foundation for understanding the complexities of different tachycardias. The second section discusses specific arrhythmia types, with an accompanying discussion of techniques for ablation. Part of the seductiveness of electrophysiology is the opportunity to offer a "cure" rather than a treatment for certain types of arrhythmias.

The book is designed for any medical professional interested in beginning a study of heart rhythms and electrophysiology, whether a cardiology fellow or electrophysiology fellow, an allied professional working in the electrophysiology laboratory, or a member of industry. One of the pleasures of electrophysiology is that these procedures require input from a number of people with different backgrounds collaborating to bring complex and specialized technology to bear on the treatment of a single patient.

There are two important topics within electrophysiology testing that can only be superficially covered in an introductory text like this. First, although implantable device therapy is an important part of electrophysiology, these devices are covered only in order to discuss the application of electrogram and ECG principles. The reader is referred to the many texts that discuss this important electrophysiology therapy in exhaustive detail. Second, new technology has become common in the electrophysiology laboratory, but complex mapping systems are only superficially discussed in this book. While these techniques are important for the advanced practitioner, it is critical to understand the basics of electrograms recorded from standard catheters before moving on to these methods. All of these tools use electrogram information and process them into color three-dimensional maps. While essential to the modern electrophysiology practice, these advanced techniques can lead one astray if the basic concepts of electrophysiology are ignored.

I am indebted to Kevin Napierkowski, who was instrumental in bringing this book from conception to reality. Nick Godwin provided the initial guidance for the project from the publishing side. I am grateful to Kate Newell from Wiley-Blackwell for supplying the gentle prodding that provides the continuous forward momentum necessary for a project such as this. I would like to thank Hugh Brazier for his clear-minded copy-editing and for ensuring that my writing conformed to the Queen's English. My staff at Mayo Clinic Florida provided important input into the figures and content of this book. In particular, Missy Weisinger obtained the necessary electrograms from our digital library for many of the illustrations. I would like to thank my family for putting up with a temporarily distracted husband and father and the many irreplaceable hours that a project like this takes. Finally, special thanks to Sumiko and Howard Kusumoto for tolerating a young "nerd" who would incessantly ask questions (what is $2 + 2 + 2 + 2$?), particularly if he was trying to get out of trouble.

Fred Kusumoto

PART 1

Electrophysiology Concepts

CHAPTER 1

Procedural issues for electrophysiologic studies: vascular access, cardiac chamber access, and catheters

Before we can discuss the relationship between electrograms and ECGs and use this information to unravel the mechanisms for arrhythmias and to design therapies, it is important to understand how procedures are performed in the electrophysiology laboratory. In general there are two types of electrophysiologic procedures: (1) electrophysiologic studies and ablation that use temporarily placed catheters to evaluate and treat arrhythmias, and (2) implantation of "permanent" cardiac rhythm devices. This book focuses on electrophysiology procedures, and our discussion of implantable devices will be limited to basic electrograms and ECGs associated with pacing therapy.

The electrophysiologic test combines standard ECG recording and electrical signals acquired from within the heart (electrograms). Electrograms are acquired using specialized thin plastic catheters that have exposed metal electrodes at the tip, connected via insulated wires to plugs that in turn can be connected to a recording device on which the signal is displayed for analysis. The catheters are placed in different cardiac chambers, and electrical signals are recorded from direct contact with the myocardium. Since electrophysiologic testing is invasive and requires vascular access, it is usually performed in a specialized cardiac suite that has fluoroscopic equipment.

Vascular access

Electrophysiologic testing and ablation procedures usually require several points for venous access, depending on operator preference, arrhythmia complexity, and patient-specific considerations. At our institution two to five separate venous sheaths are placed, depending on the case, to allow independent movement of multiple catheters. More complex arrhythmias require more simultaneous mapping points and either more venous access points or catheters with more electrodes. Smaller adults and children provide less opportunity for placing multiple sheaths safely within a single vein. Requirement for equipment such as intracardiac echocardiography necessitates additional vascular access sites.

Understanding Intracardiac EGMs and ECGs. By Fred Kusumoto. Published 2010 by Blackwell Publishing. ISBN: 978-1-4051-8410-6

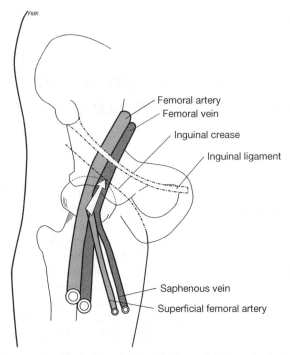

Figure 1.1 Anatomy and landmarks for cannulating the femoral vein. The femoral vein should be cannulated at the inguinal crease. Low cannulation points increase the risk of puncturing the superficial femoral artery, while high cannulation can be associated with significant bleeding into the retroperitoneal space. (Reprinted with permission from Abate E, Kusumoto FM, Goldschlager NF. Techniques for temporary pacing. In: Kusumoto FM, Goldschlager NF, eds. *Cardiac Pacing for the Clinician*, 2nd edn. New York, NY: Springer, 2008.)

The most commonly used sites for venous access are the femoral veins (Fig. 1.1). Cannulation of the femoral vein is performed by first identifying the inguinal ligament that travels from the iliac crest to the pubis. Fluoroscopically it is usually at the head of the femur. The vein should be cannulated below this landmark. The arterial pulse is palpated and a thin-wall needle is inserted at a 40° angle relative to the skin approximately 1 cm medial to the pulse. When the vein is cannulated, there will be free venous return with slight aspiration on the syringe. The syringe is removed and a guidewire is threaded through the hub of the needle into the vein. With the wire acting as a stable support, an intravascular sheath is threaded into the vein. In an adult the femoral vein can support up to three intravascular sheaths safely with minimal complications. If multiple sheaths are placed within the same femoral vein, the insertion sites are usually separated by 3–5 mm, with guidewires placed for all of the necessary access points before placing the sheaths.

Specialized long sheaths with specific shapes are often used in the electrophysiology laboratory to provide additional support and "directionality" to electrode catheters, particularly those used for ablation. At our laboratory, standard-length smaller sheaths are placed (6 French, 10 cm) and are exchanged for longer sheaths as the case unfolds. In this way, specific sheath shapes can be chosen depending on the arrhythmia type and the patient's specific anatomic characteristics.

Access from "above" has also been traditionally used in some laboratories, via the interval jugular vein or the subclavian vein. The right internal jugular vein provides a "straight line" down the superior vena cava and the right atrium. Although many laboratories still use these vascular access sites, because of patient comfort and the small but definite risk for pneumothorax, superior access sites are now generally used less frequently.

Chamber access

Correlation between fluoroscopic images and recorded electrograms is discussed in detail in Chapter 2. However, it is instructive at this time to discuss how different cardiac chambers and large veins can be reached during electrophysiologic testing. The right atrium is the easiest chamber to access, since venous return from both the inferior vena cava and superior vena cava feed directly into this chamber (Fig. 1.2). From the right atrium, catheters can be directed through the tricuspid valve to obtain recordings from the right ventricle.

Recording from the left atrium can be achieved by placing a catheter within the coronary sinus (Fig. 1.2). The coronary sinus travels near the mitral annulus and provides stable electrical signals from adjacent left atrial tissue and left ventricular tissue. Oftentimes access to the left atrium itself is required to allow

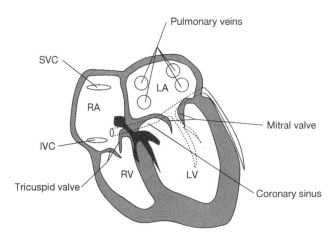

Figure 1.2 Schematic of cardiac anatomy. The coronary sinus and its venous branches provide the venous return from the coronary arterial circulation. The coronary sinus drains into the right atrium. The body of the coronary sinus travels "behind the heart" along the mitral valve annulus separating the left atrium (LA) and the left ventricle (LV). SVC, superior vena cava; IVC, inferior vena cava; RA, right atrium; RV, right ventricle.

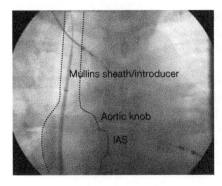

Figure 1.3 A 0.032 inch guidewire has been placed in the superior vena cava. The guidewire is then used to place a Mullins sheath/introducer into the superior vena cava. The dashed line shows the approximate course of the most septal portion of the superior vena cava and right atrium. In most cases, the Brockenbrough needle/Mullins sheath introducer will track along this course as it is slowly withdrawn. IAS, interatrial septum.

recording of electrical signals from other areas of the left atrium away from the mitral annulus

Obtaining vascular access to the left atrium is performed by puncturing a small hole through the interatrial septum. Many techniques have been developed for safe access to the left atrium, but all are a variation of the technique developed by Brockenbrough in the late 1950s. The following paragraphs describe in detail the technique used by the author for accessing the left atrium.

The Mullins sheath/introducer combination is placed in the superior vena cava at the level of the innominate vein (Fig. 1.3). After the introducer is flushed, the Brockenbrough needle is carefully inserted through the introducer. As the needle is advanced it will make two turns, one at the level of the iliac veins and the other at the level of the renal veins. The needle is advanced to a point 4–5 cm from the hub of the introducer with the inner stylet in place to prevent "snowplowing" of plastic within the lumen of the sheath. The stylet is removed and the needle is attached to a manifold that allows pressure monitoring, saline flush, and contrast injection. The Brockenbrough needle has a "pointer" that is in the same plane and direction as the needle curve. Depending on anatomy the "pointer" will be directed in the range of 4:30 to 5:30 o'clock, using a vertical clockface as a reference (Fig. 1.4). However, depending on the orientation of the heart within the body, if the interatrial septum is directed more posteriorly an orientation of 6:00 or even 8:00 is sometimes required, and if the interatrial septum is directed more anteriorly an orientation of 3:00 is required. The whole assembly (both the Mullins sheath/introducer set and the Brockenbrough needle) is slowly pulled back under fluoroscopic giuidance in the AP projection. The sheath/needle assembly will make two leftward "jumps," once at the superior vena cava/right atrium junction and then again as it falls into the fossa ovalis (Figs. 1.5, 1.6, 1.7).

At our laboratory access to the left atrium is always performed with the aid of intracardiac echocardiography using a "point and shoot" technique. Intracardiac echocardiography provides real-time information that supplements standard fluoroscopy and allows for safer entry into the left atrium. The tip of the intracardiac echocardiography catheter is placed at the fossa ovalis

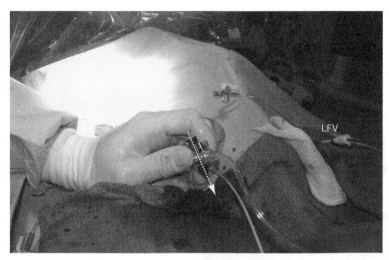

Figure 1.4 Photograph showing the orientation of the Brockenbrough needle. In this case the patient has an interatrial septum that lies more posteriorly, so a needle position of approximately 5:00 is required. Through the left femoral venous sheath (LFV) an ultrasound catheter is placed.

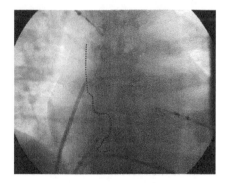

Figure 1.5 Continuation of Fig. 1.3. The wire is removed and the Brockenbrough needle is placed in the Mullins sheath/introducer, and the entire apparatus is slowly withdrawn. At this point the sheath/introducer/needle combination is still in the superior vena cava

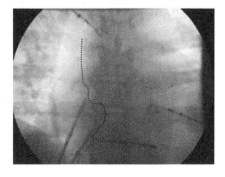

Figure 1.6 Continuation of Fig. 1.5. The entire apparatus is now at the junction of superior vena cava and right atrium.

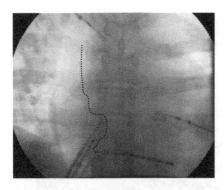

Figure 1.7 Continuation of Fig. 1.6. The sheath/introducer system will suddenly "jump" to the left as the fossa ovalis is engaged.

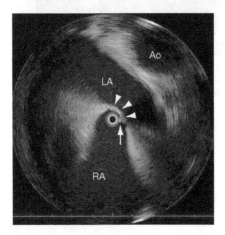

Figure 1.8 Intracardiac echocardiography is used to confirm the position of the transseptal needle within the fossa ovalis. The position of the needle can be seen as two parallel echogenic dots (arrow). The position of the intracardiac echocardiography catheter is the black circle at the middle of the image. The arrowheads show the interatrial septum. LA, left atrium; RA, right atrium; Ao, descending aorta.

and the region is explored with gentle maneuvering, and frequently a patent foramen ovale will be noted as the intracardiac echocardiography catheter is advanced into the left atrium. The superior and posterior portion of the fossa ovalis is the most common region to be probe-patent. If the fossa ovalis is not patent, or if the operator wishes to access the left atrium at a different site than the patent foramen ovale (which can sometimes be too superior and posterior to allow for maneuvering the catheter), then puncture of the interatrial septum with the needle will be required. The tip of the intracardiac echocardiography catheter can be used as a guide for the exact point the needle should be placed (Figs. 1.8, 1.9). When the needle and echocardiography catheter are placed in the same position, the echocardiographic image and the pressure tracing are evaluated. If shadowing from the catheter tip is seen within the left atrium and a left atrial pressure tracing are recorded, the Mullins introducer has already entered the left atrium through a patent foramen ovale, and the needle can be removed and a guidewire placed in the left atrium. More commonly, tenting of the interatrial septum will be observed and the pressure tracing will be dampened (Fig. 1.9). The needle is carefully extended, and with a palpable

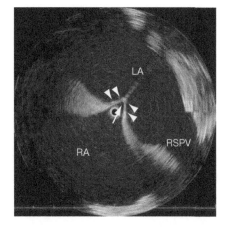

Figure 1.9 In the same patient as Fig. 1.8, as the needle or introducer is advanced, tenting of the interatrial septum (arrowheads) will be observed by intracardiac echocardiography. Artifact from the needle called shadowing can be seen within the left atrium. LA, left atrium; RA, right atrium; RSPV, right superior pulmonary vein.

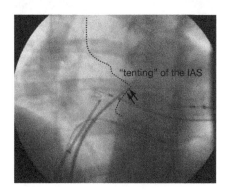

Figure 1.10 The needle is extended into the left atrium. Arrows point to the exposed needle. A palpable "pop" will frequently be felt by the operator as the left atrium is entered.

"pop" the left atrium will be entered (Fig. 1.10). This is confirmed by evaluating the pressure tracing and injection of a small amount of contrast. With experience, when the "pop" is felt the operator will learn to quickly relax any forward pressure on the needle and introducer assembly to prevent the needle from puncturing the lateral wall of the left atrium. The needle is removed and a 0.032 inch guidewire is placed into the left atrium and used as a support to advance the sheath into the left atrium (Fig. 1.11). The sheath is then used as a "passageway" to place an electrophysiologic catheter into the left atrium (Fig. 1.12). Remember that any time the left atrium is catheterized, aggressive anticoagulation is required to reduce the risk of thromboembolic complications. The use of intracardiac echocardiography has made left atrial access much safer. In fact, at our laboratory most patients are fully anticoagulated when they undergo transseptal puncture because thrombus can form quickly on catheters in some patients.

The left ventricle can be accessed using the transseptal technique, or retrogradely through the aortic valve. From a transseptal approach it is usually very

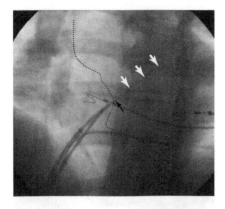

Figure 1.11 The introducer is "nosed" into the left atrium and the 0.032 inch guidewire is placed in the left atrium. The white arrows show the guidewire in the left atrium and the black arrow shows the portion of the introducer that has been placed in the left atrium.

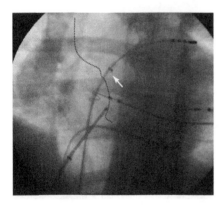

Figure 1.12 The sheath is placed into the left atrium and is used as a "passageway" for introduction of an electrophysiology catheter. The white arrow shows the portion of the sheath placed in the left atrium.

simple to advance the catheter across the mitral valve to access the left ventricle. Sometimes advancing the sheath to the mitral annulus provides support for the catheter. For the retrograde approach the femoral artery is accessed and a catheter is prolapsed across the aortic valve. Choice of the transseptal or retrograde approach depends on the operator, and on the specific regions of interest within the left ventricle.

Electrophysiologic catheters

Once sheaths are placed, specialized electrophysiologic catheters are placed within the heart. At their simplest, electrophysiologic catheters are composed of thin wires attached to electrodes located at the tip and more proximal rings insulated by plastic. Catheters will vary by the number and location of electrodes. Since electrograms are usually recorded from two adjacent electrodes, the electrode number is even, usually four, eight, or ten, although catheters with more than 20 electrodes are also available. For adult cases, catheters from

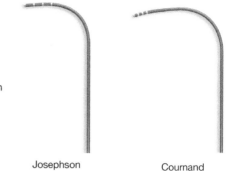

Figure 1.13 Electrophysiology catheters often come in preformed shapes that allow the clinician to manipulate the catheter to desired locations. Two commonly used fixed curved are the Josephson curve and the Cournand curve. (Courtesy of Mike Repshar, Boston Scientific.)

Josephson   Cournand

5 to 7 French are used, with the size dependent on factors ranging from cost to catheter complexity (multielectrode catheters are usually larger).

Electrophysiology catheters also come in a variety of preformed shapes depending on the intended use (Fig. 1.13). The most common shape is the "Josephson" (named after Mark Josephson, a pioneer in electrophysiology who developed the shape to allow optimal recording and manipulation characteristics for the first endovascular electrophysiologic catheters), which has a gentle curve at the tip to allow the operator to twist the catheter and guide it to the desired location. Another commonly used shape is the Cournand curve (named for André Cournand, who shared the 1956 Nobel Prize for advances in cardiac catheterization), which has a more proximal curve and a longer tip. More complex shapes include catheters designed to enter into the coronary sinus, as well as circular and basket-shaped catheters for obtaining recordings from tubular structures.

Catheters with steering capabilities have been developed by all the manufacturers, and these were an important advance, allowing catheters to be carefully moved to different positions of the heart in a reliable way. To allow even more flexibility, catheters are available with different adjustable radii, while others can be curved in both directions at a 180° angle (bidirectional).

Signal acquisition

Once catheters are placed, they can be used to record electrical activity of the heart. The two traditional methods for recording electrical signals are "unipolar" and "bipolar" (Fig. 1.14). The term "unipolar" is a misnomer, since electrical recording always requires two electrodes. However, in unipolar recoding only one electrode within the heart is used, with the second electrode being located outside the heart. The anode can be Wilson's central terminal, which uses the sum of the extremity electrodes, an electrode located within the inferior vena, or a surface electrode. When unipolar recording is used in our laboratory, most commonly an inferior vena cava electrode is used, since this configuration is less susceptible to electronic "noise" from the environment

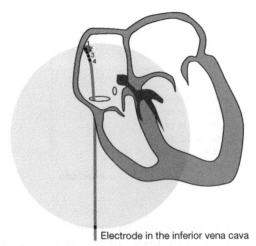

Electrode in the inferior vena cava

Figure 1.14 Schematic showing recording differences between "bipolar" and "unipolar" recordings. In bipolar recordings, the voltage differences between two electrodes placed within the heart are measured. In this schematic bipolar recording from electrodes 1 and 2 leads to a signal that reflects local activation (small circle). In unipolar recording only one electrode is within the heart and the other electrode is located outside the heart (in this case an electrode in the inferior vena cava). This leads to electrical measurement over a larger area (large circle).

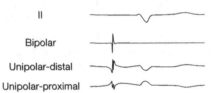

II

Bipolar

Unipolar-distal

Unipolar-proximal

Figure 1.15 Relationships between a bipolar signal recorded from electrodes 1 and 2 of a catheter placed within the right atrium and unipolar signals from the distal electrode (1) and proximal electrode (2), using an electrode in the inferior vena cava as the anode or indifferent electrode. In the unipolar signals, far-field activity from ventricular depolarization can be observed. Notice that in the bipolar electrogram, far-field signal from ventricular activity cancels out. The bipolar electrogram can be considered the sum of the unipolar signals obtained from the two intracardiac electrodes. ECG lead II is shown as a reference. Notice that the sharp high-frequency signal in the bipolar electrogram coincides with the P wave.

(other electrical equipment used in the electrophysiology laboratory). Since unipolar recording measures electrical activity over a larger distance, "far-field" activity is more commonly seen (Figs. 1.14, 1.15).

In electrophysiology laboratories, bipolar recording is most commonly used. In bipolar signals both the cathode and anode are located within the heart. Bipolar electrodes have less far-field activity since the signals cancel. This effect can be observed in Fig. 1.15. In this case unipolar signals from the proximal and distal electrodes from a catheter placed in the right atrium are shown. Notice that the unipolar signals have a broad lower-amplitude signal due to ventricular depolarization and repolarization (the waves that correspond with the QRS complex and T wave) since the signal is obtained from the electrode in the heart and Wilson's central terminal. The broad signal from ventricular depolarization is called low frequency because it is characterized by a very slow change in signal amplitude and a broader base. In a bipolar signal, the far-field ventricular signal "cancels out" and it is easier to see the effects of depolarization in a smaller region of tissue. However, unipolar recording has an important role, particularly during ablation, since the signal of interest is obtained from only the tip electrode rather than a combined signal from a distal and proximal electrode.

Catheters are connected to a "junction box" that is in turn connected to a signal amplifier, and the signal is then displayed on a recording apparatus (usually high-resolution displays and a computer system that allows signals to be selected and adjusted by the user and recorded to a hard drive or other storage medium). Within the signal amplifier, electrical signals are amplified and filtered. High-pass filters allow frequencies higher than a certain cut-off to pass through while low-pass filters allow frequencies lower than a specified frequency to pass through. Think of high-pass and low-pass filters as "shutters" that allow desired frequencies to be recorded. Notch filters are designed to remove signals from a specific unwanted frequency. In clinical use a notch filter that removes signals with a 60 Hz frequency can be used to eliminate unwanted noise from the standard alternating current that is used to power equipment used within the electrophysiology laboratory (since 60 Hz is the frequency of the alternating current).

The effects of filtering are shown in Figs. 1.16 and 1.17 for atrial and ventricular signals respectively. In Fig. 1.16, a catheter is placed in the right atrium. The top tracing shows the electrogram recorded with the high-pass filter

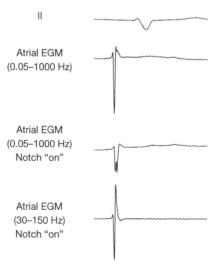

II

Atrial EGM
(0.05–1000 Hz)

Atrial EGM
(0.05–1000 Hz)
Notch "on"

Atrial EGM
(30–150 Hz)
Notch "on"

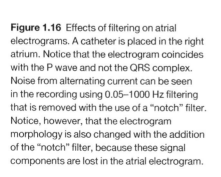

Figure 1.16 Effects of filtering on atrial electrograms. A catheter is placed in the right atrium. Notice that the electrogram coincides with the P wave and not the QRS complex. Noise from alternating current can be seen in the recording using 0.05–1000 Hz filtering that is removed with the use of a "notch" filter. Notice, however, that the electrogram morphology is also changed with the addition of the "notch" filter, because these signal components are lost in the atrial electrogram.

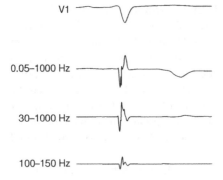

Figure 1.17 Effects of filtering on a ventricular electrogram. As the high-pass filter is increased from 0.05 to 30 Hz and finally 100 Hz, the low-frequency signal due to ventricular repolarization is gradually lost. When the low-pass filter is decreased from 1000 to 150 Hz the ventricular electrogram becomes significantly attenuated due to loss of ventricular signal content.

and low-pass filter set at 0.05 Hz and 1000 Hz respectively. Notice the regular undulating baseline due to "noise" from alternating current that is eliminated by using a notch filter (middle tracing), but the electrogram itself is also changed. In the bottom tracing the high-pass and low-pass filters are increased and decreased respectively to provide a smaller frequency recording "window," resulting in significant changes in electrogram morphology. The significant change in electrogram morphology with different filtering is one of the reasons that while electrogram timing can be measured fairly consistently it is more difficult to evaluate electrogram morphology. Figure 1.17 shows the effects of filtering on ventricular signals. Electrograms from a bipolar electrode placed in the right ventricle are shown. Since the catheter is within the right ventricle the "sharp" high-frequency signals coincide with the QRS complex. When the filters are opened widely (0.05–1000 Hz), a high-frequency signal associated with ventricular depolarization is observed along with a lower-frequency signal due to ventricular repolarization that coincides with the T wave. Since T waves generally have a frequency of 0.05–10 Hz, as the high-pass filter is increased from 0.05 to 30 and finally 100 Hz, the wave due to ventricular repolarization becomes attenuated. The frequency of ventricular activity is usually between 50 and 150 Hz, with some additional higher-frequency components, so that as the low-pass filter is decreased, the ventricular signal becomes attenuated. These two figures illustrate the important effects of filtering on the electrograms that are recorded during electrophysiologic studies.

CHAPTER 2

Fluoroscopic anatomy and electrophysiologic recording in the heart

The number and positioning of electrophysiologic catheters will depend on the type of arrhythmia and the aim of electrophysiologic testing. For example, in a patient with ventricular tachycardia in which the clinician intends to map and potentially ablate the cause for ventricular tachycardia, more catheters will be placed in the ventricle and generally no catheters will be placed in the atria. However, in electrophysiology studies where the type of arrhythmia is unknown, many clinicians will start with catheters placed in the right atrium, straddling the tricuspid valve, in the right ventricle, and in the coronary sinus (Fig. 2.1). These four positions allow relatively complete evaluation of all electrical regions of the heart using only venous access.

Fluoroscopic anatomy

Since electrophysiology catheters are predominantly placed in right-sided structures it is important to review right-sided anatomy. The important features of right-sided cardiac anatomy are shown in Fig. 2.2. Venous return from the body enters the right atrium from the inferior vena cava and the superior

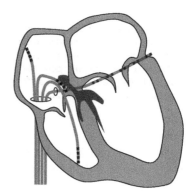

Figure 2.1 Schematic of the chambers of the heart and standard catheter positions often used for baseline electrophysiologic studies.

Understanding Intracardiac EGMs and ECGs. By Fred Kusumoto. Published 2010 by Blackwell Publishing. ISBN: 978-1-4051-8410-6

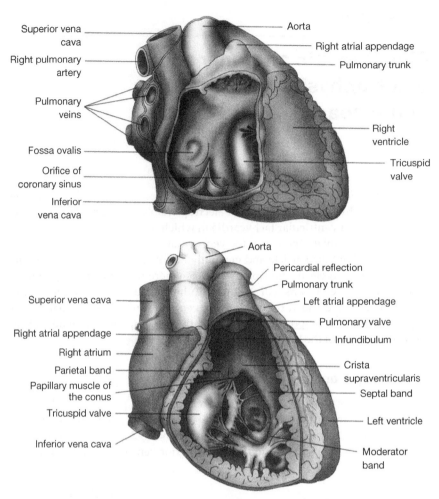

Figure 2.2 Anatomic drawings of the right-sided cardiac chambers. *Top:* On the right atrial side blood returns to the heart via the superior and inferior venae cavae. *Bottom:* On the right ventricular side, blood flows in through the tricuspid valve and out through the pulmonary valve to the lungs. (Reprinted with permission from Kusumoto FM. Cardiovascular disorders: heart disease. In: McPhee SJ, Lingappa VR, Ganong WF, eds. *Pathophysiology of Disease*, 5th edn. New York, NY: McGraw-Hill, 2003.)

vena cava. Blood flows across the tricuspid valve, and with ventricular contraction takes a "U-turn" and travels out through the pulmonary valve and into the pulmonary arteries. The coronary sinus empties into the inferior and septal right atrial wall near the tricuspid valve. The body of the coronary sinus straddles the left atrium and left ventricle and is not seen in this view of the right atrium and right ventricle, but it is shown in Fig. 2.3 as it travels epicardially between the left atrium and the left ventricle. The coronary sinus

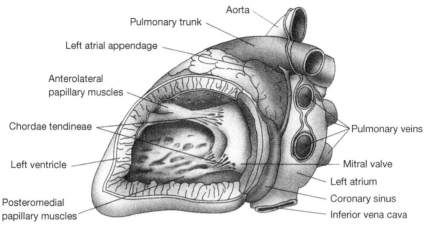

Figure 2.3 Anatomic drawing of the left-sided chambers. The coronary sinus travels epicardially between the left atrium and left ventricle. It receives venous branches that return blood from the left ventricle and left atrium. (Reprinted with permission from Kusumoto FM. Cardiovascular disorders: heart disease. In: McPhee SJ, Lingappa VR, Ganong WF, eds. *Pathophysiology of Disease*, 5th edn. New York, NY: McGraw-Hill, 2003.)

is the way blood from the coronary circulation returns to the heart. In Fig. 2.4, standard catheter positions are superimposed on the anatomic drawings. In this example the positions of quadripolar catheters placed in the right ventricle, right atrium, and straddling the tricuspid valve (for His bundle recording) are shown. A fourth catheter (a decapolar catheter) is sometimes placed within the coronary sinus.

Since anatomic landmarks cannot be seen directly during electrophysiology procedures, fluoroscopy has been traditionally used to aid catheter positioning within the heart. Fluoroscopy uses an x-ray source coupled to an x-ray image intensifier and video camera that allows continuous x-ray images to be observed. It is important for the student to understand the anatomic position of catheters with standard fluoroscopic imaging. Generally fluoroscopic images are obtained in the right anterior oblique (RAO) and the left anterior oblique (LAO) orientations (Fig. 2.5).

In the RAO view the mitral and tricuspid valves are perpendicular to the image, so the atria are located on one side and the ventricles on the other. By convention in most laboratories the atria are shown on the left side of the image and the ventricles are on the right side. In the RAO projection the right-sided chambers are "in front" and the left-sided chambers are "in back." Figure 2.6 shows an RAO view with electrophysiology catheters in position. Quadripolar catheters are located in the right atrium (RA), right ventricle (RV), and straddling the right atrium and right ventricle (His). A decapolar catheter in the coronary sinus is "going away" from the viewer, since the left-sided chambers and mitral valve are behind the right-sided chambers and the tricuspid valve in this view.

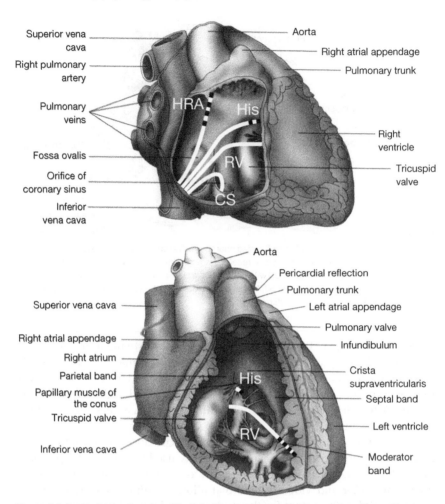

Figure 2.4 Anatomic drawings from Fig. 2.2 with superimposed catheters placed in positions commonly used for electrophysiologic testing: high right atrium (HRA), His bundle position (His), right ventricle (RV), and coronary sinus (CS). (Adapted from Kusumoto FM. Cardiovascular disorders: heart disease. In: McPhee SJ, Lingappa VR, Ganong WF, eds. *Pathophysiology of Disease*, 5th edn. New York, NY: McGraw-Hill, 2003.)

In the LAO view the mitral and tricuspid valves are "on face" and can be represented as full circles that are side-by-side. By convention the tricuspid valve is shown on the left and the mitral valve on the right. Figure 2.7 shows the LAO view from the same patient as in Fig. 2.6. Notice that the decapolar catheter in the coronary sinus is directed toward the right along the inferior border of the coronary sinus. The His bundle catheter and right ventricular catheters are "coming out" of the picture plane toward the viewer since the right ventricle is "in front" of the right atrium. In the anterior–posterior (AP) view the valve plane is at an angle to the image plane. Figure 2.8 shows an AP fluoroscopic image of the same patient as in Figs. 2.6 and 2.7. In this view the

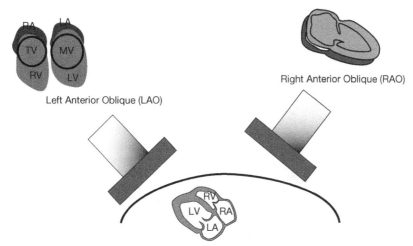

Right Anterior Oblique (RAO)

Left Anterior Oblique (LAO)

Figure 2.5 Schematic of standard fluoroscopic angles obtained during an electrophysiologic study. In the left anterior oblique (LAO) angle one looks at the heart "down a two-barreled shotgun." The orifices of the mitral valve and tricuspid valve are directly seen, with the atria "behind" and the ventricles "in front" of the valve plane. In the right anterior oblique (RAO) position, the mitral and tricuspid valve plane is oriented perpendicular to the image plane and the atria and ventricles are to the left and right sides of the image respectively.

Figure 2.6 Fluoroscopic image in the right anterior oblique (RAO) position. The right atrium is oriented to the left and the right ventricle is to the right. Quadripolar catheters placed in the superior portion of the right atrium (RA), in the right ventricle (RV), and straddling the right atrium and right ventricle (His) can be seen. Notice that the tricuspid valve (TV) and mitral valve (MV) are perpendicular to each other. A decapolar catheter placed into the coronary sinus (CS) is "traveling away" from the viewer.

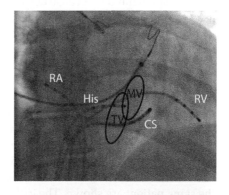

Figure 2.7 Fluoroscopic image from the same patient as in Fig. 2.6 in the left anterior oblique (LAO) position. Now the coronary sinus catheter (CS) can be seen traveling along the inferior portion of the mitral valve (MV). The right ventricular (RV) and His bundle catheters are "coming out" of the image plane towards the viewer, and the right atrial catheter (RA) is directed away from the viewer. IVC, inferior vena cava; SVC, superior vena cava; TV, tricuspid valve.

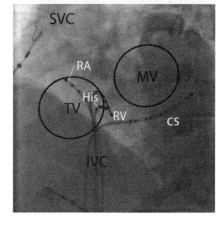

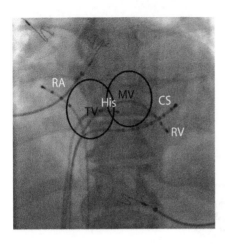

Figure 2.8 Fluoroscopic image of the same patient in the anterior–posterior (AP) orientation. In this view the mitral and tricuspid valve plane is at an angle to the image plane. Notice that the spine runs down the middle of the image. Abbreviations as in Fig. 2.6.

mitral valve and tricuspid valve partially overlap, and the spine now runs down the middle of the image. Notice that in the LAO view the spine is located to the right (since it is more posterior) and in the RAO view the spine is located on the left side of the image (again because the spine is more posterior).

It is important that the relationship between the RAO and LAO views is always kept in mind to reconstruct a three-dimensional "picture" of a patient's heart. In the RAO view the atria and ventricles are "side-by-side," so it is easy to distinguish between atrial and ventricular catheters. However in this orientation it is impossible to determine whether catheters are in the left-sided or right-sided chambers, since they are superimposed. Similarly, in the RAO orientation it is impossible to determine whether a catheter is located on the free-wall or the septal side of a given chamber. Conversely, in the LAO position it is easy to determine whether catheters are in the left- or right-sided chambers or whether a catheter is located septally or at the free wall, but since there is significant overlap of the right atrium and right ventricle and the left atrium and left ventricle it is often difficult to determine the anterior and posterior orientation of catheters. For example, in Fig. 2.9, LAO and RAO images of the same patient are shown. The catheters are in the same position except for the catheter placed in the right atrium (arrow). Although the catheters are related similarly to the lateral wall (dotted line) in the RAO images, one can see from the LAO images that in the images on the left the catheter is pointed anteriorly toward the right atrial free wall and in the images on the right the catheter is pointed posteriorly toward the interatrial septum. Understanding the relationship between RAO and LAO images is particularly important when catheters are placed in the left-sided chambers. In Fig. 2.10, a decapolar catheter is placed in the right atrium along the lateral wall. This is why the catheter extends toward the left (away from the spine) in the LAO view. A quadripolar catheter has been placed in the left atrium via a transseptal puncture. This can best be seen in the LAO view, where the catheter is closer to the spine and is above the coronary sinus catheter.

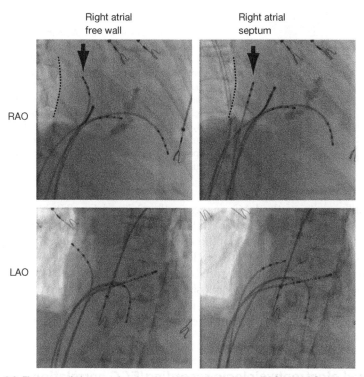

Figure 2.9 Fluoroscopic images showing the relationship between RAO and LAO views. In the left column, a catheter is placed at the free wall of the right atrium (arrow) and in the right column the catheter has been rotated and directed toward the interatrial septum (arrow). In the RAO views, the relationship between the catheter tip and the free wall (dotted line) is similar since the RAO image provides very little information on whether a catheter is located at the septum or free wall. Differentiating between right atrial free-wall and septal positions can be easily determined in the LAO projection. RAO: Right anterior oblique; LAO: Left anterior oblique

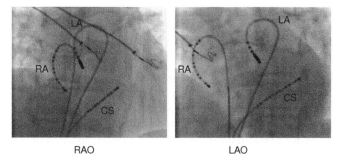

Figure 2.10 Fluoroscopic images in the RAO and LAO views. In this case a decapolar catheter is located in the right atrium (RA), a second decapolar catheter is in the coronary sinus (CS), and a quadripolar catheter has been placed in the left atrium (LA) using a transseptal technique. The LAO view is required to help differentiate between left atrial and right atrial positions. RAO: Right anterior oblique; LAO: Left anterior oblique

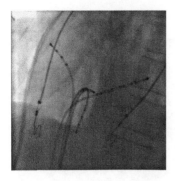

Figure 2.11 A true LAO view (60°) in the patient from Fig. 2.9. In Fig. 2.9 even with an LAO angle of 40° the curve of the His bundle catheter and the wide spacing between the four electrodes can be seen. A true LAO position, with no overlap of the mitral and tricuspid valves, can be determined by elimination of the curve in the His bundle catheter with the four electrodes located "on top of each other." This finding suggests that the His catheter is truly perpendicular to the imaging plane. In this case, because of rotation of the heart within the body, a true LAO position required an angle of 60°. LAO: Left anterior oblique.

Finally, compare the LAO images in Fig. 2.7 and Fig. 2.9. Notice that in Fig. 2.9 the four electrodes of the His bundle catheter are "spread apart," which suggests that the catheter is not directed perpendicular to the imaging plane. In this patient a standard LAO angle of 40° did not eliminate overlap of the mitral and tricuspid valves. A true LAO view (60°) is shown in Fig. 2.11. This patient had significant kyphoscoliosis, with the apex of the heart directed very posteriorly, and a steeper angle was required to achieve a true LAO view. This example shows how the His bundle catheter can be used to determine whether a true LAO view has been obtained.

Normal electrophysiologic recording/ECG correlation

Now that we have defined the location of our catheters by fluoroscopy we can use the electrical signals obtained from surface ECG leads and the electro-physiologic catheters to provide insight into the normal activation of the heart. Throughout this discussion it is important to emphasize that electrical signals obtained from endocardial catheters provide important but complementary information to the surface ECG, and electrograms should always be considered in the context of ECG signals.

With this in mind, when analyzing intracardiac electrograms it is a good habit to always look at the simultaneous surface ECG. At first, the ECG signals recorded during electrophysiologic testing are hard to interpret because of the difference in sweep speeds (Fig. 2.12). Normally the ECG is recorded at 25 mm/second, but intracardiac signals are evaluated at faster sweep speeds: 100 mm/second or higher, depending on the signals of interest. In Fig. 2.12, at a sweep speed of 25 mm/second, the individual waves of the surface ECG are easy to distinguish, but the intracardiac electrograms are "too smooshed" to evaluate. In order to evaluate these complex signals, analysis of intracardiac electrograms require higher sweep speeds to "spread out" individual signals from different catheters. At higher sweep speeds the P wave and T wave are harder to pick out, but the QRS complex is still reasonably easy to see. However, with practice, evaluation of surface ECG characteristics at higher sweep speeds will become second nature. Experienced laboratory personnel

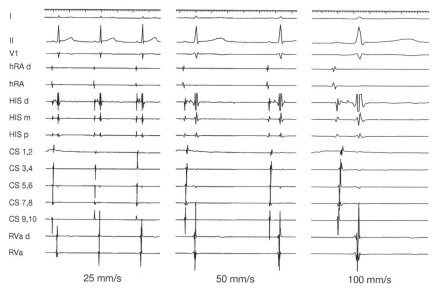

25 mm/s   50 mm/s   100 mm/s

Figure 2.12 Effect of different sweep speeds on surface ECG and intracardiac electrograms. As the sweep speed is increased from 25 mm/second to 50 mm/second, and finally 100 mm/second, the P wave becomes harder to appreciate in the surface ECG (leads I, II, and V_1) but the intracardiac electrograms recorded from the high right atrium (HRA), His bundle region (His), coronary sinus (CS), and right ventricle (RV) become easier to interpret as the signals from different chambers become more "spread out."

will be able to identify P waves and T waves, differentiate between normal appearing and wide QRS complexes, and evaluate specific morphology characteristics of the QRS complex and the P wave.

The electrograms obtained from our patient with fluoroscopic images (Figs. 2.6, 2.7, 2.8) are shown in Figs. 2.13 and 2.14. When analyzing intracardiac electrograms themselves it is important to first determine how the signals are displayed. Unlike 12-lead ECGs, there is no standard display format for recording intracardiac electrograms. This is not surprising, given the variety of catheters with different numbers of electrodes that can be placed or moved to multiple regions of the heart. Within our laboratory, different electrophysiologists will choose different display formats, based on personal preference. In general, each catheter is given a "name," usually based on location. RA (right atrium), His (His bundle region), RV (right ventricle), and CS (coronary sinus) are used in our laboratory. In many laboratories, the signals are arranged in a manner that mimics normal cardiac depolarization, with the right atrial signals on top followed by the His bundle and the coronary sinus, with the right ventricular signal on the bottom. For each catheter the signals obtained from each electrode pair can be displayed by electrode numbers or by location.

Figure 2.13 shows a typical baseline recording. Surface ECGs are generally placed highest to encourage initial analysis of the surface ECG before evaluating EGMs. In this example lead II and V_1 from the surface ECG are shown.

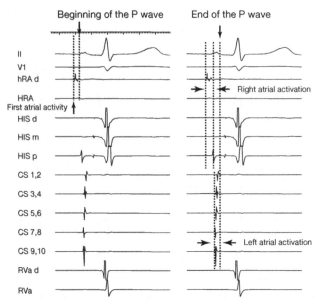

Figure 2.13 Baseline electrograms emphasizing the pattern of atrial activation. The first recorded atrial electrogram occurs before the onset of the P wave in the catheter positioned at the high right atrium. Right atrial activation is generally complete when an atrial signal is recorded in the His catheter that straddles the right atrium and right ventricle along the septal wall. Left atrial activation occurs after right atrial activation, and the latest atrial signal is recorded in the distal electrodes of the coronary sinus catheter (CS 1,2).

A quadripolar catheter placed in the superior portion of the right atrium is labeled HRA (for high right atrium), with the bipolar signal from the distal two electrodes (1 and 2) labeled as HRA d and the bipolar signal from the proximal electrodes (3 and 4) left without a label. The next three tracings are from a quadripolar catheter placed in the region of the His bundle straddling the right atrium and right ventricle with the catheter tip just past the tricuspid valve. The three tracings are labeled HIS d (distal electrodes 1 and 2), HIS m ("mid" electrodes 2 and 3), and HIS p (proximal electrodes 3 and 4). The next five tracings are from the coronary sinus catheter (CS), with the specific electrode pairs listed (1,2; 3,4; 5,6; etc. – with electrodes listed from distal to proximal as 1 through 10). Finally, the last two tracings are from a catheter placed in the right ventricular apex (RVa), with the recordings from electrode 1 and 2 listed as distal (d). Again, it is important to emphasize that different laboratories will use different catheters and display formats depending on preference and study type, and it is imperative to note "what catheters are where" before spending any time on EGM analysis.

Normally, the sinus node is the fastest pacemaker of the heart and "drives" depolarization of the rest of the heart. Since the sinus node is located in the superior portion of the right atrium near the junction between the superior vena cava and the right atrium, the first electrogram is usually recorded in a catheter located in this region (Fig. 2.13). Notice that the bipolar signal from this position is actually recorded earlier than the inscription of the P wave. The amount of tissue initially depolarized is too small to be recorded on the surface by the standard ECG. The wave of depolarization travels to the interatrial septum, where an atrial signal can be observed in the catheter that straddles the right atrium and right ventricle. Left atrial activation recorded by the catheter placed in the coronary sinus can then be observed. Notice that right atrial activation occurs during the initial portion of the P wave and left atrial activation during the terminal portion of the P wave. This activation pattern is a consequence of the location of the sinus node, high in the right atrium near the junction of the superior vena cava. Not surprisingly, the latest atrial signal is recorded in CS 1,2, which is located at the lateral free wall of the left atrium (examine LAO fluoroscopy in Fig. 2.7 and notice that the distal tip of the coronary sinus catheter is located the greatest distance away from the right atrial catheter).

Once the atrial septum is depolarized, the atrioventricular (AV) node is activated (Fig. 2.14). The AV node is too small to produce a measurable electrogram with our usual clinical tools because the upstroke of the action potential of the AV node is slower, being dependent mainly on opening of Ca^{2+} channels. Once the AV node is activated the wave of depolarization travels rapidly over the bundle of His. A discrete His signal can be recorded, since this tissue uses Na^+ channels for depolarization. Thus conduction through the AV node can be estimated by measuring the interval between the atrial signal measured and the initial deflection of the His bundle potential. This interval is called the *AH interval*. The interval between the His bundle and the first deflection noted on the surface ECG is called the *HV interval*, and it represents conduction from

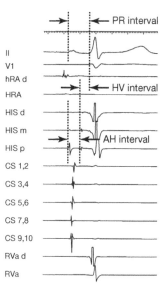

Figure 2.14 Baseline activation emphasizing atrioventricular conduction. The AH interval measures the time interval from initial atrial activation near the interatrial septum to initial activation of the His bundle. This interval provides an excellent surrogate for conduction through the AV node. The interval from initial activation of the His bundle to initial ventricular depolarization observed on the QRS is called the HV interval and provides an estimate for the conduction time for the His–Purkinje system.

the His bundle through the left and right bundles to initial ventricular activation by Purkinje fibers. Thus atrioventricular conduction can be seen to have two components, a longer AH interval due to slow AV nodal conduction that starts at some point within the P wave and ends at the His bundle and a faster conduction period that represents the last portion of the PR interval. The normal AH interval varies with autonomic tone but usually ranges from 50 to 140 ms. Changes in the AH interval are common with changes in autonomic tone. His–Purkinje tissue has very little autonomic input, and consequently the HV interval will generally be stable during an electrophysiology procedure. The normal value for the HV interval in adults ranges from 30 to 55 ms.

On the ECG the PR interval is measured from the beginning of the P wave to the beginning of the QRS (Fig. 2.14). The PR interval then has three components: right atrial conduction, AV node conduction, and His bundle and distal bundle conduction. Notice that the AV node conduction is the largest portion of the PR interval. Although prolongation of the PR interval could be due to delay in any of the three components, the largest contributor is AV node conduction.

The ventricles are depolarized almost simultaneously via the His–Purkinje system, so the QRS complex is usually less than 0.12 seconds (Fig. 2.15). Notice, however, that the ventricular signal measured within the coronary sinus is measured at the end of the QRS as this portion. Sometimes a discrete potential due to depolarization of the right bundle will be recorded just before the ventricular signal (Fig. 2.16). The right bundle potential can sometimes be confused with the His signal, but will normally occur < 30 ms before the ventricular electrogram, and there will be no accompanying atrial signal at a site where a right bundle potential is recorded. As will be discussed in Chapter 4, it can

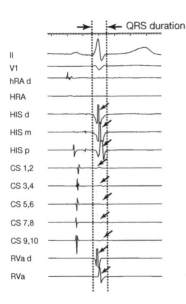

Figure 2.15 Ventricular depolarization normally occurs over a very short period of time, particularly when once considers the relative size of the cardiac chambers (think of the relative widths of P waves and the QRS complex). Earliest ventricular signals are usually observed in the His bundle and right ventricular catheters, because these are usually placed along the interventricular septum. The inferior and posterior portions of the left ventricle (seen as low-amplitude low-frequency signals in CS 3,4 and CS 5,6) are usually the latest site of ventricular activation in normal conditions.

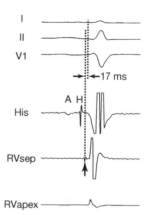

Figure 2.16 Intracardiac electrograms showing the difference between a His bundle signal and a right bundle potential. The His signal has a discrete isoelectric period before ventricular activation due to the time required for Purkinje tissue activation. In contrast, a right bundle potential will be observed slightly before the QRS with a potential–QRS interval of less than 30 ms. In this case the interval between the right bundle potential and the initial portion of the QRS complex is 17 ms.

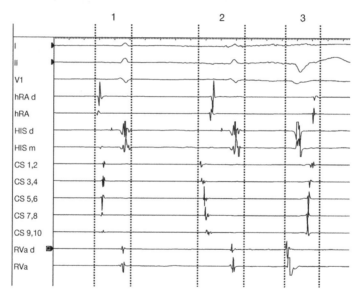

Figure 2.17 Three consecutive beats with different causes. Beat 1: sinus rhythm with initial electrogram recorded in the right atrial catheter. Beat 2: premature atrial contraction due to a left-sided focus with earliest atrial signal recorded in the distal coronary sinus electrodes, with normal atrioventricular conduction and ventricular depolarization. Beat 3: a premature ventricular contraction characterized by initial depolarization noted in the right ventricle with retrograde activation of the atria via the AV node. This is why atrial activation appears to emanate from the region near the coronary sinus os at electrodes 9,10 of the coronary sinus catheter.

sometimes be difficult to differentiate between a right bundle potential and a potential due to activation of the distal His bundle.

Intracardiac electrograms provide valuable detail for evaluating premature beats. In Fig. 2.17 electrograms from three consecutive heart beats are shown. In beat 1, the patient has a normal sinus beat. Atrial activation starts in the right atrium and ends in the left atrium. A normal His bundle signal can be observed. In beat 2, atrial activation starts in the distal coronary sinus, with left atrial depolarization preceding right atrial depolarization. A His bundle signal is recorded, followed by a subsequent QRS due to normal ventricular depolarization. From the atrial activation pattern, one can logically guess that beat 2 represents a premature atrial contraction arising from the lateral wall of the left atrium. Beat 3 represents a premature ventricular contraction. Although the QRS complex is hard to evaluate at this sweep speed, the first upstroke of ventricular depolarization can be seen in the distal two electrodes of the right ventricular catheter. The QRS complex is not preceded by atrial depolarization. In addition, notice that atrial activation after the premature ventricular contraction can be seen in the right atrial and coronary sinus catheters. Notice that the first atrial signal is observed at the os of the coronary sinus (CS 9,10). This activation is probably due to retrograde activation via the AV node. Thus from these three consecutive beats one can see the utility of intracardiac electrograms for comprehensive beat-to-beat analysis of cardiac depolarization: sinus rhythm in the first beat, a premature atrial contraction arising from the left atrium for the second beat, and a premature ventricular contraction leading to retrograde atrial activation via the AV node for the third beat.

CHAPTER 3

Programmed stimulation

Once catheters are in place, comprehensive electrophysiologic testing requires baseline evaluation of intracardiac electrograms followed by analyzing the effects of electrical stimulation (pacing) of the heart (Table 3.1). The cardiac responses to pacing provide important insight into the electrophysiologic properties of the heart, and pacing may induce arrhythmias. Once a tachycardia is induced, single or multiple stimuli are delivered during tachycardia at specific points during the cardiac cycle to help determine the mechanism of the arrhythmia.

Programmed stimulation should be performed systematically. It is critical for a clinician to have some idea of a patient's clinical diagnosis, based on history or preparatory test results such as the baseline ECG, ECG during symptoms, or imaging studies (echocardiography, computed tomography, cardiac catheterization, etc.). However, balanced with this, the clinician should always keep an "open mind," and it is essential that programmed stimulation be performed in a repeatable and methodical manner. At our institution we perform atrial overdrive pacing, premature atrial stimulation, ventricular overdrive pacing, and ventricular extrastimulation in almost every patient referred for electrophysiologic study, regardless of the specific clinical indication for the electrophysiology study.

Table 3.1 Overview of the components of an electrophysiology study.

Baseline evaluation (intervals)
Pacing • Atrial (constant intervals, premature extrastimuli) • Ventricular (constant intervals, premature extrastimuli)
Evaluation of tachycardia • Activation pattern in tachycardia (atrial and ventricular) • Initiation • Termination • Response to timed extrastimuli

Understanding Intracardiac EGMs and ECGs. By Fred Kusumoto. Published 2010 by Blackwell Publishing. ISBN: 978-1-4051-8410-6

Baseline pacing

Basic principles
Pacing is performed by choosing the chamber to be paced and confirming capture of cardiac tissue. For most stimulators the pulse width is fixed (usually 2 ms) and the output is adjusted to capture myocardial tissue. In Fig. 3.1, pacing from the high right atrium is performed. At 0.5 mA the pacing stimuli do not capture atrial tissue. As the output is increased to 0.8 mA partial capture in a 2 : 1 pattern is achieved. Finally, as the output is increased to 1.0 mA, 1 : 1 capture is present. In this case the pacing "threshold" is 1 mA. Pacing during programmed stimulation is generally set at 3.0 mA or twice threshold. If greater current is required to reliably capture the cardiac tissue, it is usually prudent to change the position of the catheter to obtain a site with a better threshold.

Figure 3.1 shows pacing performed from the high right atrium, so atrial activation at the His bundle area and the left atrium (as represented by the coronary sinus) electrograms have the same general temporal relationship. Notice, however, that the pattern of activation in the coronary sinus electrograms (ellipses) is different than during sinus rhythm. This can occur because of two possibilities. First, pacing is performed at a right atrial site that is near but not at the sinus node, which leads to a different pattern of left atrial activation. Second, with more rapid atrial activation the pattern of atrial activation can change due to the development of regions of tissue that exhibit slower conduction or refractoriness.

Finally, an issue on pacing nomenclature in the electrophysiology laboratory should be discussed here. Although with implanted pacemakers that pace at constant rates it is easier to think of pacing rates and beats per minute, in the electrophysiology laboratory, where pacing is often not performed at constant rates and premature extrastimuli are delivered, it is easier to think of intervals between pacing stimuli. So delivering constant stimuli at 600 ms intervals is pacing at a rate of 100 beats per minute, at 500 ms intervals the pacing rate is 120 beats per minute, and at 400 ms intervals the pacing rate is 150 beats per minute.

Atrial overdrive pacing
Pacing from the atria is used to determined atrioventricular conduction properties, usually by using the ventricular response to stimuli to evaluate the atrioventricular conduction system as a "black box."

Figure 3.1 (*opposite*) Determining the pacing threshold. *Top*: Pacing (*) at 0.5 mA does not result in atrial capture. Although one is tempted to think that the second pacing stimulus resulted in atrial capture, the astute reader will note that the baseline sinus rate is unchanged and the relationship between the pacing stimulus and the atrial electrograms is coincidence. *Middle:* The pacing output is increased to 0.8 mA and every other pacing stimulus results in atrial capture (2 : 1 capture). *Bottom:* The pacing output is increased to 1.0 mA and now every pacing stimulus results in atrial capture.

No Capture

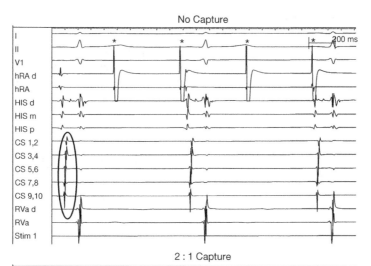

2 : 1 Capture

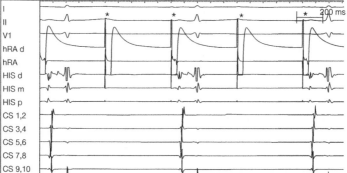

1 : 1 Capture

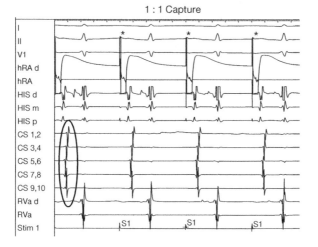

An example of atrial pacing in a patient at progressively shorter cycle lengths is shown in Figs. 3.2, 3.3, and 3.4. For all three figures, catheters are positioned in the right atrium, right ventricle, His bundle position, and coronary sinus, as shown in Figs. 2.1, 2.4, 2.6, and 2.7 in Chapter 2. In Fig. 3.2, with atrial pacing at a cycle length of 600 ms (paced rate of 100 beats per minute), there is a

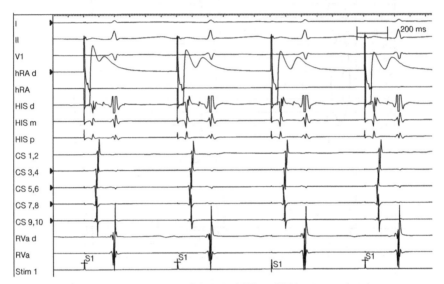

Figure 3.2 Atrial pacing at a constant cycle length of 600 ms (100 beats per minute)

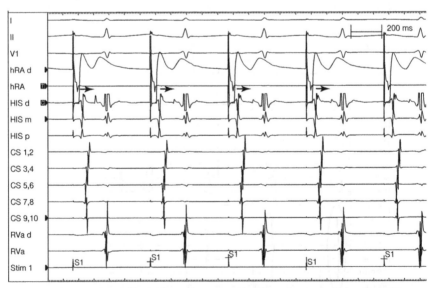

Figure 3.3 Same patient as Fig. 3.2 but with more rapid atrial pacing at a cycle length of 450 ms. The relationship between atrial stimulation and ventricular response remains 1 : 1, but due to normal delay in the AV node the AH interval increases (arrows).

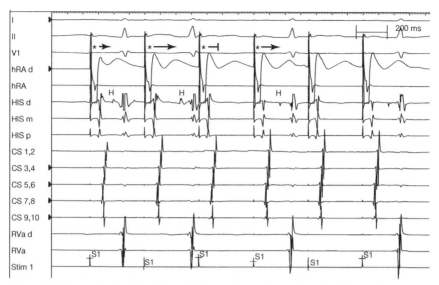

Figure 3.4 Same patient as Figs. 3.2 and 3.3 but pacing at shorter intervals (350 ms). At this pacing rate (about 170 beats per minute) the relationship between atrial stimulation and ventricular response is no longer 1 : 1. The interval between atrial electrogram and His bundle signal (H) increases until block in the AV node occurs (an atrial electrogram without a His signal).

1 : 1 atrial and ventricular relationship. In Fig. 3.3, stimulation frequency is increased to a cycle length of 450 ms (pacing rate of 133 beats per minute), and the AH interval increases due to the normal decremental conduction properties of the AV node. Notice that the HV interval and the QRS complex remain the same, confirming that conduction through the His–Purkinje system and ventricular activation remain unchanged even with more rapid atrial stimulation. In Fig. 3.4, the stimulation interval is shortened to 350 ms (pacing rate of 171 beats per minute) and now the relationship between atrial stimulation and ventricular response is no longer 1 : 1. With each pacing stimulus there is progressive prolongation of the AH interval until there is a dropped beat. Since the pacing stimulus is associated with an atrial electrogram but no His (H) electrogram, one can ascertain that the site of block is within the AV node.

Gradual prolongation of AV node conduction is often called *Wenckebach block* in honor of Karl Wenckebach, who described this phenomenon in the 1800s by careful evaluation of the jugular venous pulsation and the peripheral pulse. A schematic illustrating the development of AV Wenckebach is shown in Fig. 3.5. The cycle length at which the relationship between atrial stimulus and ventricular response is no longer 1 : 1 is called the atrioventricular blocked cycle length or AVBCL. The development of AV block at fast atrial rates is a normal response called *decremental conduction*, which "protects" the ventricles from rapid rates. A nice analogy is to think of the AV node as a site where a four-lane road shrinks to two lanes before returning to four lanes. Although this can cause headaches on the highway it helps reduce the flow of cars in the

Progressive AV delay

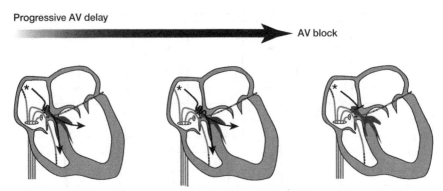

AV block

Figure 3.5 Schematic of atrioventricular block with pacing. As the pacing cycle length is decreased, gradual delay and ultimately block will develop in atrioventricular conduction. The cycle length at which the atrial : ventricular relationship is no longer 1 : 1 is called the atrioventricular blocked cycle length or AVBCL. The gradual prolongation of atrioventricular block is called AV Wenckebach. Atrioventricular block usually develops in the AV node, because of the electrophysiologic properties of the AV node, but in some cases can develop at the His bundle or below the His bundle. When block occurs at these tissues below the AV node, the Wenckebach phenomenon is usually not observed.

region beyond the constriction. This strategy is used on freeway onramps in some metropolitan areas, where traffic lights are used to regulate flow onto the freeway and reduce traffic congestion. Clinically this important effect is most commonly observed when a patient develops atrial fibrillation. Although atrial fibrillation leads to rapid ventricular rates, the situation would be far worse if the AV node conducted every fibrillatory depolarization to the ventricles. The AVBCL provides information on the "robustness" of atrioventricular conduction. Development of AV Wenckebach block at rapid paced rates is normal. However, development of AV Wenckebach block during normal sinus rhythm or at slow paced rates suggests the presence of AV nodal disease, as discussed more fully in the next chapter.

Atrial premature stimulation

In addition to pacing the heart at a constant rate, comprehensive electro-physiologic testing also requires providing single or multiple premature beats. To understand the effects of premature beats, it is important to understand one of the fundamental electrophysiological properties of cardiac tissue: refractoriness.

The concept of refractoriness is illustrated in Fig. 3.6. As an extrastimulus is brought in earlier and earlier, initially another normal action potential will be produced. However, at some point, as activation occurs earlier, fewer Na^+ channels are available for activation and the phase 0 upslope becomes less steep and the conduction velocity slows. If the extrastimulus is delivered still earlier, then at some point there are no Na^+ channels that can be activated and no matter what the strength of the stimulus a second action potential cannot

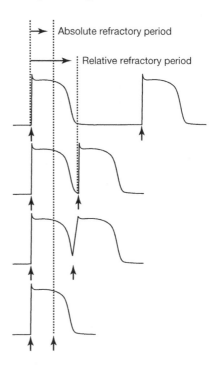

Figure 3.6 Concept of refractoriness. As an extrastimulus is more closely coupled, at first a subnormal phase 0 upstroke occurs (relative refractoriness) and then a point is reached where an extrastimulus does not produce a phase 0 upstroke (absolute refractoriness).

be produced. The interval in which no action potential can be produced is called the absolute refractory period, and the period in which abnormal activation occurs is called the relative refractory period. The concept of refractoriness is important in understanding electrophysiology. The refractory period provides a rough estimate for the action potential duration and, as will be seen later, it is relative differences in refractoriness that are responsible for the development of reentry, which is the most common mechanism for tachyarrhythmias.

Traditionally a train of eight beats at a cycle length faster than the spontaneous sinus rate is delivered (this is called the drive cycle length), and the ninth stimulus is varied by gradually decreasing the interval between the eighth and ninth beat. In this way the refractory properties of cardiac tissue can be methodically evaluated. The stimuli within the drive train are usually called S_1 and the premature beat is called S_2. Any additional premature beats are called S_3, S_4, etc. This can be a source of some confusion, since the first premature beat is called S_2 and the second premature beat is called S_3.

An example of a normal response to progressively earlier premature atrial extrastimuli is shown in Figs. 3.7, 3.8, and 3.9. Figure 3.7 shows the introduction of a single premature atrial extrastimulus (S_2). In response to this premature beat the interval between the stimulus and the atrial electrogram recorded in the His bundle recording is the same. There is slight prolongation of the AH interval due to delayed conduction within the AV node. Notice that the HV

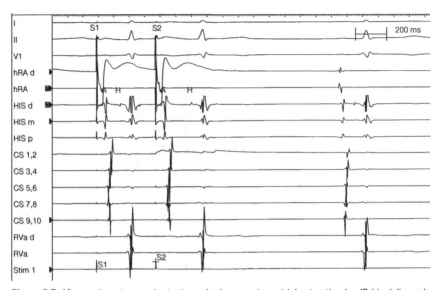

Figure 3.7 After pacing at a constant rate, a single premature atrial extrastimulus (S_2) is delivered at a coupling interval of 380 ms (as measured by the interval between S_1 and S_2). The response to the atrial extrastimulus is described in the text. A, atrial electrogram; H, His bundle electrogram.

Table 3.2 Recognition of delayed conduction in response to atrial extrastimuli.

Tissue	Response
Atrial tissue	Prolongation of the interval between the stimulus and the atrial electrogram
AV node	Prolongation of the interval between atrial electrogram and His electrogram
His–Purkinje system	Prolongation of the interval between the His electrogram and the initial deflection in the QRS complex
Ventricular activation	Widening of the QRS interval

interval remains constant and ventricular activation remains unchanged. So, expressed in simple terms, the premature beat was associated with normal conduction through atrial tissue, delayed conduction in the AV node (due to the AV node being relatively refractory), normal conduction through the His–Purkinje system, and normal ventricular activation (Table 3.2).

In Fig. 3.8, the premature atrial extrastimulus is delivered at a shorter coupling interval (320 ms), and in this case the atrial premature beat results in an atrial electrogram but no subsequent His signal or QRS complex. In this case depolarization within the AV node has blocked because the absolute refractory period of the AV node has been reached. Clinically, the term *effective*

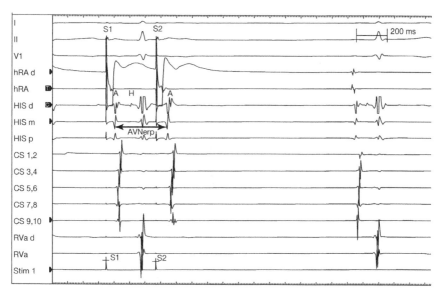

Figure 3.8 With an earlier premature atrial extrastimulus, coupled at 320 ms, depolarization is blocked in the AV node, resulting in an atrial electrogram with no His bundle recording. The interval between successive atrial electrograms is 330 ms, so this would be the AV node effective refractory period (AVNerp). A, atrial electrogram; H, His bundle electrogram.

refractory period is used to describe the coupling interval where depolarization no longer propagates through the tissue of interest. The refractory period of the AV node is calculated by measuring the interval between successive atrial electrograms in the His bundle recording. The astute reader will notice that the stimulus–atrial electrogram interval has also increased for the extrastimulus, suggesting that relative refractoriness of atrial tissue may also be present.

In Fig. 3.9, an even earlier atrial extrastimulus is delivered, and in this case the stimulus does not result in atrial depolarization because atrial tissue is completely refractory at the stimulation site (no atrial electrograms: the "stimulus cannot propagate from catheter tip to adjacent atrial tissue"). The interval between S_1 and S_2 would be a measure of the atrial refractory period. Figure 3.10 schematically illustrates the changes in intervals associated with refractoriness of different tissues in response to atrial extrastimuli. If atrial tissue becomes relatively refractory, then the interval between the stimulus and the atrial electrogram will increase (if the atrial tissue is completely refractory a stimulus without an atrial signal will be observed, as shown in Fig. 3.9). If the premature extrastimulus encroaches on AV nodal refractoriness the AH interval will increase. Finally, refractoriness of infraHisian tissue will result in prolongation of the interval between the His electrogram and the QRS (Table 3.3).

The response to extrastimuli will vary depending on the relative refractoriness of the different types of tissue. For example, if the refractory period of atrial tissue is longer than the refractory period of AV nodal tissue, the clinician

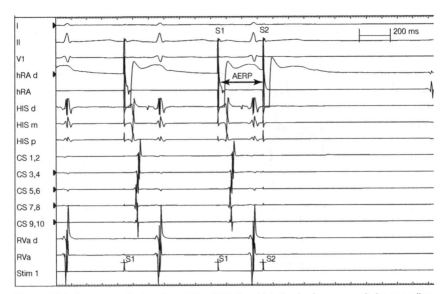

Figure 3.9 In the same patient as Figs. 3.7 and 3.8, the atrial stimulus is now coupled even earlier (280 ms). In this case, because atrial tissue at the stimulation site is refractory, the stimulus produces no atrial depolarization or electrogram. In this case the interval between S_1 and S_2 (280 ms) would be the atrial effective refractory period (AERP).

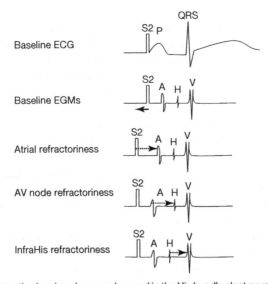

Figure 3.10 Schematic showing changes observed in the His bundle electrograms when the relative refractory periods of different tissues are reached. The top two tracings show the surface ECG and His bundle electrograms at baseline. As the S_2 is made more premature, if atrial tissue becomes relatively refractory an increase in the interval from stimulus to atrial electrogram will be observed. The most common response is encroachment on refractoriness of AV nodal tissue, resulting in prolongation of the AH interval. Rarely, the S_2 will encroach on refractoriness of infraHisian tissue, which would result in prolongation of the interval between the His electrogram and the QRS.

Table 3.3 Calculation and characteristics of refractory periods for different types of cardiac tissue.

Refractory period	Signal observed
Atrioventricular node effective refractory period (AVNERP)	Premature atrial stimulus, atrial depolarization, but no His signal and no ventricular depolarization
Atrial effective refractory period (AERP)	Premature atrial stimulus without atrial depolarization
Ventriculoatrial refractory period (VAERP)	Premature ventricular stimulus, ventricular depolarization but no atrial activity
Ventricular effective refractory period (VERP)	Premature ventricular stimulus with no ventricular depolarization

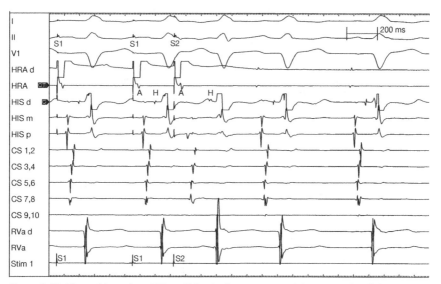

Figure 3.11 After a drive train at 600 ms (S$_1$) a single premature atrial extrastimulus (S$_2$) is delivered at a coupling interval of 270 ms. The extrastimulus results in an atrial electrogram, His potential, and QRS with normal prolongation of the AH interval.

might "run into" atrial refractoriness before he encounters refractoriness of AV nodal tissue. In order to evaluate AV node refractoriness the electrophysiologist takes advantage of a property of atrial and ventricular tissue: with earlier coupling intervals, refractory periods decrease. By using first and second extrastimuli (S$_2$ and S$_3$), the first extrastimulus can be used as a "conditioning" impulse to shorten the refractory period of atrial tissue. In this way more closely coupled atrial activation can be used to measure the refractory period of "downstream" tissue such as the AV node. An example of this phenomenon is shown in Figs. 3.11, 3.12, and 3.13. In Fig. 3.11, at a coupling interval of 270 ms the extrastimulus (S$_2$) yields an atrial electrogram, His electrogram (H),

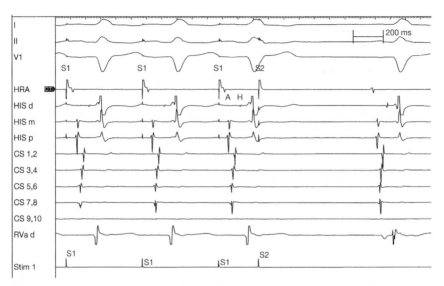

Figure 3.12 In the same patient as Fig. 3.11, a slightly more premature atrial extrastimulus coupled at 260 ms does not lead to an atrial electrogram. The interval between the two stimuli (260 ms) would be the atrial effective refractory period.

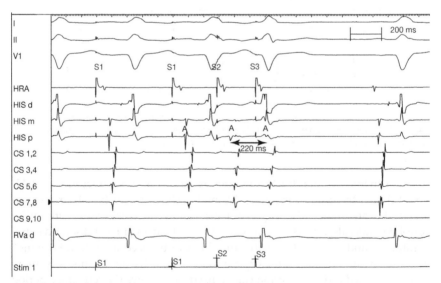

Figure 3.13 In order to evaluate the properties of the AV node in the same patient, two atrial extrastimuli are delivered, the first (S_2) with a coupling interval of 280 ms and the second (S_3) at 220 ms. This results in two atrial electrograms but no conduction through the AV node associated with the S_3. The AV node effective refractory period can now be calculated at 220 ms.

and QRS complex with normal decrement in the AV node. In Fig. 3.12, the atrial premature beat is coupled at a slightly shorter interval of 260 ms and in this case the premature extrastimulus does not capture atrial tissue, so the atrial effective refractory period would be calculated to be 260 ms. However, since atrial refractoriness was reached before AV node refractoriness, the clinician cannot assess the electrophysiologic properties of the AV node. In order to shorten the atrial refractory period, two atrial extrastimuli are provided, as shown in Fig. 3.13. A first extrastimulus (S_2) is delivered at a coupling interval of 280 ms (above the atrial effective refractory period), and a second extrastimulus (S_3) delivered at a coupling interval of 220 ms leads to an atrial electrogram but no subsequent His electrogram. In this case, the first extrastimulus acts as a "conditioning impulse" that allows a second extrastimulus to be delivered, and AV block occurs. In this case the AV node effective refractory period would be calculated to be 220 ms: the distance between the atrial electrograms from the S_2 and S_3 as recorded in the His electrodes. As a corollary to this point, it is important to realize that the effective refractory period of atrial tissue is dynamic. In fact, refractory periods of all tissues will change depending on conditions. For example, refractory periods of most cardiac tissues will decrease with infusion of a beta-agonist such as isoproterenol.

A commonly observed normal response to atrial extrastimuli is a single extra atrial beat that is due to reentry within atrial tissue (Figs. 3.14, 3.15). In Fig. 3.14, a premature atrial extrastimulus results in an additional beat,

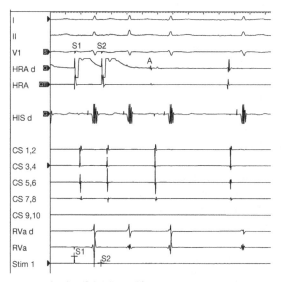

Figure 3.14 After an extrastimulus (S_2) delivered from a catheter placed in the high right atrium (HRA), an additional atrial beat is produced. The additional atrial beat results in a QRS complex and normal atrioventricular conduction. The earliest atrial electrogram (A) for the extra beat is in the HRA catheter, suggesting that the region within the high right atrium was the source for the premature beat.

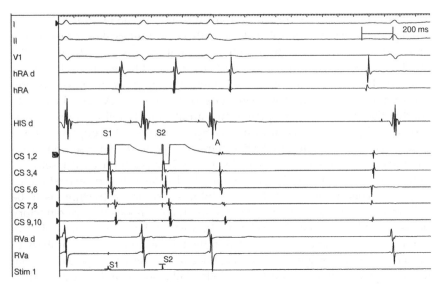

Figure 3.15 During pacing from the distal coronary sinus (notice that the stimulus artifact is seen on CS 1,2 electrodes), an atrial extrastimulus (S_2) results in a premature atrial beat with the earliest atrial signal (A) observed in the distal coronary sinus electrodes (CS 1,2). In this case, because the AV node is refractory, the premature beat does not result in a QRS complex.

with earliest atrial activation observed in the high right atrial catheter. This additional beat is probably due to interatrial reentry and is a commonly observed normal response with atrial extrastimulation. In Fig. 3.15, during pacing from the coronary sinus, an atrial extrastimulus results in an additional premature beat that is earliest in the left atrium. In contrast to the additional beat produced in Fig. 3.14, in this case atrial depolarization does not lead to a QRS complex because the AV node is refractory. Although the concept of reentry will be covered in depth in later chapters on tachycardia (Chapters 5 and 6), for the purposes of this discussion it is sufficient to note that the premature atrial extrastimulus encounters regions of refractory tissue and an extra set of atrial electrograms will be produced.

Ventricular overdrive pacing

The heart can also be paced from the ventricle, to determine whether an arrhythmia can be induced and for evaluation of the retrograde conduction properties of the AV node and His bundle. It is important to remember that the AV node and His bundle provide a "two-way street" for communication between the atria and the ventricles. Since the sinus node is the fastest intrinsic pacemaker, conduction occurs from atria to ventricles. Artificially pacing the ventricle at a more rapid rate leads to retrograde conduction through the His bundle and AV node. At slower rates the atrial response to ventricular stimuli will remain 1 : 1 (Fig. 3.16), but with more rapid ventricular pacing VA conduction block will occur (Fig. 3.17). The interval where ventricular stimuli do

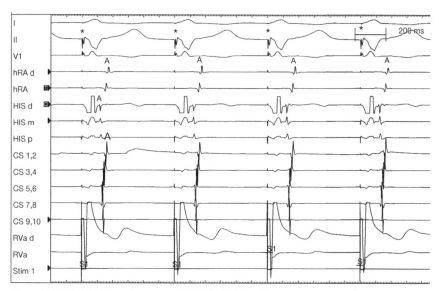

Figure 3.16 Ventricular pacing at a cycle length of 600 ms (100 beats per minute). For every ventricular paced beat (*) an atrial signal is observed (A). Notice that the first atrial signal is observed in the His bundle electrograms, because the atria are being activated retrogradely via the AV node.

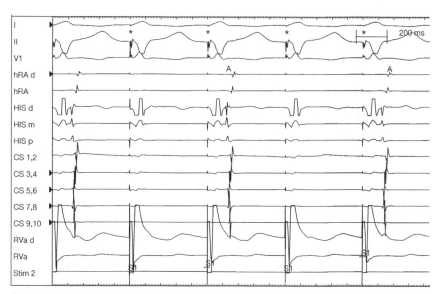

Figure 3.17 In the same patient as Fig. 3.16, when the ventricular pacing cycle length is decreased to 500 ms, 2 : 1 retrogade block in the AV node develops. This interval is called the ventriculoatrial blocked cycle length or VABCL.

not result in a 1 : 1 atrial response is termed the ventriculoatrial blocked cycle length or VABCL. Notice that in Figs. 3.16 and 3.17 the first atrial electrogram is observed in the His bundle electrograms, followed by the coronary sinus, with the high right atrium last. This pattern of "low–high" atrial depolarization is consistent with retrograde activation of the atria via the AV node.

Normally pacing is performed from the right ventricular apex. In some cases, pacing from the right ventricular outflow tract is performed, and very rarely left ventricular pacing can be used. In some cases pacing from near the His bundle provides valuable information for determining the mechanism of supraventricular arrhythmias. The morphology of the QRS complex can provide clues for the site of pacing. Pacing from the right ventricular apex leads to a QRS complex with a left bundle branch block morphology. Remember that with left bundle branch block the ventricles are activated sequentially, with depolarization of the right ventricle preceding depolarization of the left ventricle. The QRS morphology also provides clues for specific locations within the right ventricle. Pacing from the right ventricular outflow tract will lead to a QRS with an inferior axis in the inferior leads (II, III, and aVF), while pacing from the inferior apex (a common position for permanent leads used in implanted pacemakers) will lead to a QRS with a superior axis. It is important to evaluate the QRS complex associated with pacing. First, if no QRS is seen ventricular capture is not present. Second, the QRS should always have a left bundle branch block morphology in lead V_1 (wide negative QRS). If a wide positive QRS complex in lead V_1 is noted, the catheter should be evaluated with fluoroscopy, since a right bundle branch block morphology with ventricular pacing suggests that the left ventricle is being depolarized before the right ventricle, and this might represent the first sign of left ventricular pacing due to inadvertent positioning of the catheter within one of the venous branches of the coronary sinus, catheter perforation of the right ventricular free wall (with the catheter coming to rest on the left ventricular epicardium), or, less likely, perforation of the interventricular septum.

Ventricular premature stimulation

Premature ventricular stimulation can help determine refractory periods for ventricular tissue and the ventriculoatrial conduction system. In Fig. 3.18, a premature ventricular stimulus (S_2) is delivered at a coupling interval of 600 ms and ventriculoatrial conduction is still present: an atrial electrogram is observed in response to the ventricular stimulation. When the ventricular stimulus is delivered slightly earlier (Fig. 3.19) an atrial signal is not observed, because one of the tissues connecting the ventricles to the atria (His bundle, AV node) is now refractory. This interval is the ventriculoatrial refractory period, because it can be very difficult to identify a retrograde His deflection and confirm the exact site of block. When the ventricular stimulus is delivered even earlier and the stimulus does not produce ventricular depolarization (a QRS complex), then the ventricular effective refractory period has been reached.

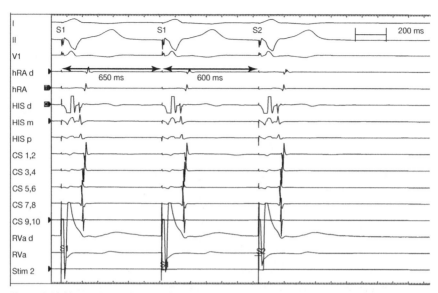

Figure 3.18 Ventricular pacing is performed with a drive cycle length of 650 ms, and a premature ventricular stimulus coupled at 600 ms is delivered. The premature ventricular stimulus is associated with retrograde AV node conduction.

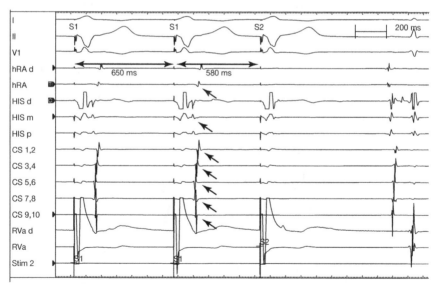

Figure 3.19 In the same patient as Fig. 3.18, when the coupling interval for the ventricular extrastimulus is decreased to 580 ms, retrograde atrial activation (arrows) is not observed with the ventricular premature extrastimulus due to retrograde block in the AV node. The interval between S_1 and S_2 (580 ms) would be the ventriculoatrial effective refractory period (VAERP).

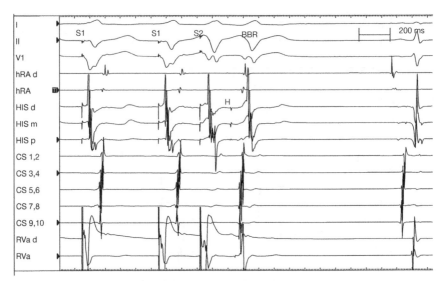

Figure 3.20 Bundle branch reentry associated with a ventricular extrastimulus. After a premature extrastimulus (S$_2$), an additional wide QRS complex beat due to bundle branch reentry (BBR) is produced. Notice the His bundle signal (H) in the His bundle recordings.

One common response to ventricular extrastimulation is a single beat of bundle branch reentry (Fig. 3.20). In this case, the premature ventricular contraction blocks retrogradely in the right bundle but the wave of depolarization travels across the ventricular septum and backwards up the left bundle. If the right bundle has recovered, the wave of repolarization enters the right bundle in the correct direction and an extra QRS complex will be observed. Since the ventricle was activated solely by the right bundle, the QRS will have a wide left bundle branch block pattern with a negative QRS complex noted in V$_1$. In addition, because the His bundle is activated retrogradely, a His bundle signal will be observed prior to the QRS complex. A schematic of the events associated with bundle branch reentry is shown in Fig. 3.21.

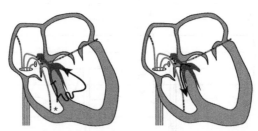

Figure 3.21 A schematic showing the events associated with bundle branch reentry. The premature ventricular extrastimulus blocks retrogradely in the right bundle but the wave of depolarization travels slowly across the interventricular septum and travels backwards up the left bundle. The wave of depolarization reenters the right bundle and leads to an additional QRS complex that is wide and has a left bundle branch block morphology because the right ventricle is depolarized before the left ventricle.

A single beat of bundle branch reentry is common. Sustained bundle branch reentry is very uncommon, and this arrhythmia will be discussed more fully in Chapter 14.

Pacing during tachycardia

If tachycardia is induced, pacing is performed during the arrhythmia to help determine the arrhythmia mechanism and to determine the anatomic components of the tachycardia. Specific pacing maneuvers will be discussed in the subsequent chapters, but a general discussion on how extrastimuli are delivered in tachycardia is reasonable here.

To deliver paced beats at specific points during the tachycardia it is important to understand the concept of *sensing*. Remember that intrinsic cardiac activity produces an electrical signal that can be recorded from surface electrodes (electrocardiogram) or from intracardiac electrodes (electrograms). The electrical signal measured at these points can be used for timing of extrastimuli delivered during tachycardia.

All stimulators and recording systems used in the electrophysiology laboratory allow the user to choose which channel to sense from. In most cases the user wishes to sense ventricular activity, so generally one of the surface ECG leads is used. The S_1 is then used to sense rather than to pace and the S_2 interval is gradually decreased. In Fig. 3.22, a narrow complex with a rate of 130 beats per minute is present. Earliest atrial activation appears to be in the His proximal electrodes. The stimulator is set to sense and deliver an S_2 ventricular

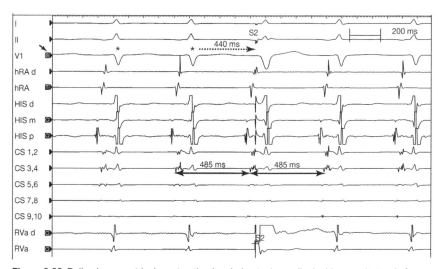

Figure 3.22 Delivering a ventricular extrastimulus during tachycardia. In this case, instead of timing the S_2 to the drive cycle, the S_2 is timed to the intrinsic QRS. The QRS complexes are sensed (*) and a ventricular extrastimulus is delivered at a programmed interval (440 ms) resulting in a slight change in the QRS morphology, but the tachycardia remains unaffected.

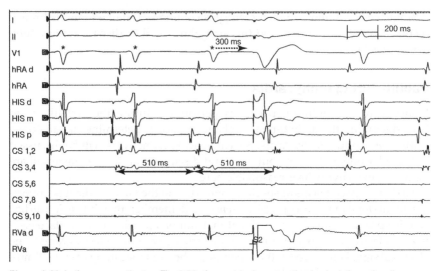

Figure 3.23 In the same patient as Fig. 3.22, the ventricular extrastimulus is delivered earlier (300 ms). This results in a wide QRS complex from ventricular pacing but the tachycardia is still not affected (the cycle length of the tachycardia has increased slightly to 510 ms).

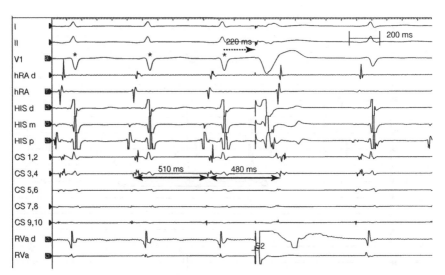

Figure 3.24 Now the extrastimulus is delivered 220 ms after the sensed QRS complex, and in this case the paced beat interacts with the tachycardia, leading to a single shorter cycle length. This change in cycle length must have occurred in response to the ventricular extrastimulus.

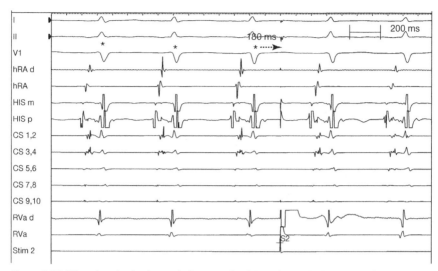

Figure 3.25 When the stimulus is coupled even earlier (180 ms), ventricular capture does not occur because the ventricle is refractory.

stimulus at a programmed interval. In this case surface lead V_1 is chosen to sense, as denoted by a small S (single headed arrow). Sensed QRS complexes are counted (*), and after the eighth sensed beat a ventricular stimulus is delivered at a programmed interval. Notice that at this first longer coupling interval a slight change in the QRS morphology is noted but the tachycardia is unaffected (double headed arrows). In Fig. 3.23, the ventricular stimulus is delivered earlier, resulting in a completely different QRS complex, but the tachycardia remains unaffected. However, in Fig. 3.24 a still earlier ventricular stimulus is delivered, and in this case the atrial signal occurs earlier, thus proving that the stimulus has "interacted" with the tachycardia. In Fig. 3.25, with an earlier ventricular stimulus (coupled to 180 ms), the ventricular tissue is refractory and a QRS is not produced. This would be the ventricular effective refractory period. The response of a supraventricular tachycardia to ventricular stimuli provides clues for identifying the tachycardia mechanism, and this will be discussed in detail in Chapter 5.

Summary

It should be clear that the comprehensive electrophysiology test has a number of essential components that can answer a variety of questions, as summarized in Table 3.4. The components of an electrophysiology study will depend on the clinical question that needs to answered. For example, in a patient with documented supraventricular tachycardia atrial and ventricular pacing including

Table 3.4 Components of a comprehensive electrophysiologic study.

Evaluation	Components	Questions
Baseline recording	Evaluation of the sequence of atrial activation	Does atrial activation proceed in the normal manner from right to left and "high–low?"
	Evaluation of atrioventricular conduction	Are the PR, AH, and HV intervals normal?
	Evaluation of ventricular activation	Is the QRS normal morphology and duration?
Atrial pacing	Evaluation of atrioventricular conduction	At what cycle length does atrioventricular block occur?
		When atrioventricular block does occur, where is the site of block?
	Evaluation of sinus node function	What is the response of the sinus node after pacing?
Atrial extrastimuli	Atrioventricular refractory periods	What are the refractory periods of different types of tissue?
	Atrial refractory periods	
Ventricular pacing	Evaluation of ventriculoatrial conduction	At what cycle length does ventriculoatrial block occur?
		When ventriculoatrial block does occur, where is the site of block?
Ventricular extrastimuli	Ventriculoatrial refractory periods	What are the refractory periods of different types of tissues?
	Ventricular refractory periods	
Evaluation of arrhythmias	Method of induction	How was the arrhythmia induced (atrial pacing, ventricular pacing, extrastimuli)?
	Sequence and activation pattern of atrial and ventricular depolarization during tachycardia	What is the temporal pattern of atrial and ventricular activation?
		What is the pattern of ventricular and atrial depolarization?
	Response to stimuli	How does the tachycardia respond to pacing protocols?

one or two extrastimuli will be used. In contrast, an electrophysiology study that is being performed to evaluate risk of ventricular arrhythmias in a patient with coronary artery disease may not involve any atrial pacing but may use aggressive ventricular stimulation protocols with up to three ventricular extrastimuli.

CHAPTER 4

Bradycardia

Although invasive electrophysiologic testing is generally used for assessment of tachycardia, it also has an important role in the evaluation of patients with bradycardia. Bradycardia can be caused by sinus node dysfunction (no P waves) or atrioventricular block (P waves without an accompanying QRS).

Sinus node dysfunction

In sinus node dysfunction, the sinus node does not generate depolarization at a normal rate. The manifestations of sinus node dysfunction are quite diverse. Clinically, patients can present with lightheadedness, syncope, dizziness, fatigue, or exercise intolerance. The ECG manifestations are equally diverse and include sinus bradycardia, sinus pauses and alternating episodes of brady-cardia and tachycardia (brady-tachy syndrome).

The electrophysiologic findings for sinus node dysfunction are helpful but not diagnostic. It is important to note that none of the indications for permanent pacing actually uses information from electrophysiologic testing.

One of the most common parameters used for evaluation of sinus node function is the *sinus node recovery time* (SNRT). The atria are paced at a constant cycle length for 30 seconds and pacing is then abruptly stopped. The interval from the last pacing stimulus to the first spontaneous electrogram that arises from the vicinity of the sinus node (the high lateral right atrium) is the SNRT. The concept is that the longer the sinus node takes to recover the more abnormal sinus node function is. Since depolarization of the sinus node will vary by pacing rate, the SNRT is measured with different pacing rates. The maximum recorded time is used as the best measure of sinus node automaticity. The SNRT is usually corrected to the intrinsic sinus rate by calculating the difference between the maximal SNRT and the sinus cycle length. The normal value of the corrected SNRT is usually less than 550 ms. An example of an abnormal SNRT is shown in Fig. 4.1. With atrial pacing at a cycle length of 400 ms, with sudden cessation of pacing it takes 2.2 seconds for sinus node function to return. Notice that there is a single junctional beat that occurs before the sinus node recovers. In this case the SNRT would be 2200 ms and the corrected SNRT would be 1800 ms (2200 − 400 ms). Other less commonly used tests are

Understanding Intracardiac EGMs and ECGs. By Fred Kusumoto. Published 2010 by Blackwell Publishing. ISBN: 978-1-4051-8410-6

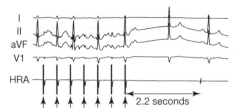

Figure 4.1 Sinus node recovery time (SNRT). The high right atrium (HRA) is paced at a cycle length of 400 ms for 30 seconds (small arrows). After cessation of pacing sinus node automaticity returns after a delay of 2.2 seconds. (Reprinted with permission from Stevenson IH, Sparks PB, Kalman JM. Sinus node dysfunction. In: Kusumoto FM, Goldschlager NF, eds. *Cardiac Pacing for the Clinician*, 2nd edn. New York, NY: Springer, 2008.)

the sinoatrial conduction time and direct measurement of the sinus node action potential. These techniques are not usually employed at most electrophysiology laboratories, and neither will be covered here.

The true clinical value of electrophysiologic testing for evaluating sinus node function is unknown but probably limited. Prolonged ECG monitoring (event recorders and implantable loop recorders) rather than invasive electrophysiologic testing is a more fruitful method for diagnostic evaluation in patients suspected of having symptomatic sinus node dysfunction.

Atrioventricular conduction block

The ability to record activation of the His bundle played a fundamental role in the development of invasive electrophysiologic evaluation. The relationship between the His bundle recording and other cardiac signals (the intracardiac atrial electrogram and the QRS complex) provides insight into the site of AV block and the refractory properties of tissue connecting the atria and the ventricles.

Baseline evaluation

On the surface ECG, the PR interval provides a rough estimate for atrioventricular conduction. An abnormal PR interval is defined as greater than 0.22 seconds. As discussed in the previous chapter, electrophysiologic testing allows evaluation of the relative conduction properties of the tissues that make up the atrioventricular conduction axis: AV node, His bundle, and infraHisian conduction tissue (bundles). The AH interval is quite variable, since it will at least in part be due to changes in sympathetic and parasympathetic tone. In contrast, the HV interval is not generally affected by autonomic input, and normal values are more easily defined. The normal HV interval is usually between 35 and 55 ms. An HV interval > 55 ms is generally considered abnormal, although moderate prolongation of the HV interval (55–70 ms) has not been shown to be associated with higher risk for developing complete heart block. An HV interval > 100 ms would be classified as extremely abnormal. In

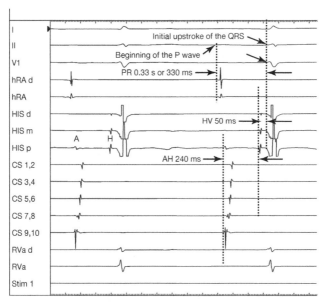

Figure 4.2 Electrograms from a patient with a prolonged PR interval. The patient has a markedly prolonged PR interval of 0.33 seconds (330 ms). Intracardiac electrograms reveal that the predominant reason for this increase is prolongation of the AH interval 240 ms.

fact, finding an HV interval > 100 ms in a patient with syncope should make the clinician seriously consider implantation of a permanent pacemaker.

Figure 4.2 shows the baseline electrograms from a man with first-degree AV block noted on an ECG. Although the P wave can sometimes be difficult to see at higher sweep speeds, the PR interval is extremely prolonged at 0.33 seconds or 330 ms. The intracardiac electrograms reveal that the reason for the prolonged PR interval is significant prolongation of the AH interval, confirming that the patient has disease in the AV node. The HV interval is within normal limits at 50 ms, which suggests that conduction over the His–Purkinje system remains normal. Now examine the electrograms in Fig. 4.3. Again, first-degree AV block is present (PR 0.28 seconds). However, in this case there are two His signals, one recorded in the mid portion of the His catheter (H1) and a later deflection recorded in the distal His electrodes (H2). This patient has intraHisian delay. It can be very difficult to distinguish between potentials due to His bundle activation and right bundle activation. In general, in the absence of distal disease beyond the right bundle, the interval between the right bundle potential and the QRS complex should be less than 30 ms. In this case the interval between the H2 potential and the QRS complex is 50 ms in the presence of a normal QRS complex, making a multicomponent His signal more likely. Interestingly, in asymptomatic patients, the presence of intraHisian delay does not appear to bode a worse prognosis. When there are multiple components to the His bundle electrograms, the HV interval is measured from the first His

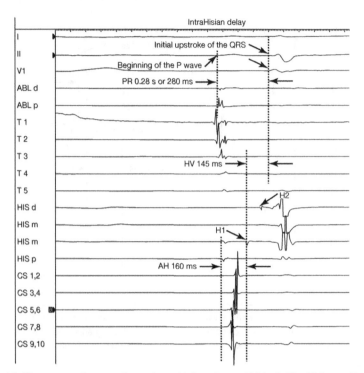

Figure 4.3 Electrograms from another patient with first-degree AV block. The PR interval is prolonged (0.28 seconds), but in this case the AH interval is within normal limits (160 ms) but there is significant intraHisian delay with multiple His signals recorded. The HV interval is measured from the first His signal.

signal. Finally, Fig. 4.4 shows a patient with a normal PR interval (0.19 seconds), but the intracardiac electrograms reveal a markedly prolonged HV interval of > 100 ms, which is indicative of infraHisian disease. Note that of the three cases, the last patient, with the shortest PR interval, is actually at the highest risk for developing severe symptomatic bradycardia.

Electrophysiology testing is very useful for evaluating asymptomatic patients with second-degree AV block (the P wave to QRS relationship is no longer 1 : 1) (Fig. 4.5). Block in the AV node can have a relatively slow progression and, since the site of block is within the AV node, if complete heart block develops the patient may complain of fatigue but often does not have syncope because of automaticity at one of the AV nodal sites below the level of block. Conversely, if complete infraHisian block develops, the patient is dependent on automaticity from ventricular tissue, which is notoriously unreliable. For this reason evidence of infraHisian block, even in an asymptomatic patient, is an indication for permanent pacing. Figure 4.6 is from an asymptomatic patient with 2 : 1 AV block. The presence of type I second-degree AV block is usually indicative of block within the AV node, while type II block is associated with infraHisian block. With 2 : 1 block it is more difficult, and

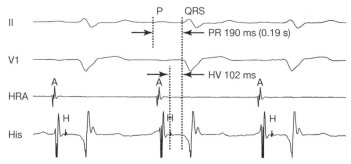

Figure 4.4 Intracardiac electrograms reveal a prolonged HV interval (102 ms), which is evidence for infraHisian disease despite the presence of a PR interval within normal limits (< 0.20 seconds).

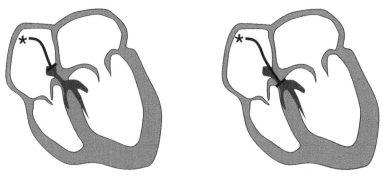

Block in the AV node
•Atrial signal without His signal or QRS

Block below the His bundle
•Atrial and His signals without a QRS

Figure 4.5 Schematic showing the use of intracardiac electrograms for evaluating the site of block. If block occurs within the AV node, when an atrial paced beat is associated with a dropped QRS complex no His signal will be observed. If block occurs in infraHisian tissue, the atrial beat with the dropped QRS complex will have an associated His recording.

sometimes impossible, to determine the site of block. In this case, the intra-cardiac electrograms reveal that the site of block is in infraHisian tissue. The nonconducted P wave is associated with both an atrial electrogram and a His electrogram. The patient was referred for permanent pacing therapy.

AV blocked cycle length

Remember that the AV blocked cycle length is the pacing rate at which AV conduction stops having a 1 : 1 relationship. The normal AV blocked cycle length ranges from 350 to 500 ms, but it is very dependent on autonomic tone. From our previous discussion, it is important to identify the presence of block below the His bundle. The site of atrioventricular block can be determined by electrophysiologic testing. If the block is occurring within the AV node an atrial signal without a His bundle signal will be seen (Fig. 4.5). If block is infraHisian a His bundle electrogram will be observed but no subsequent QRS

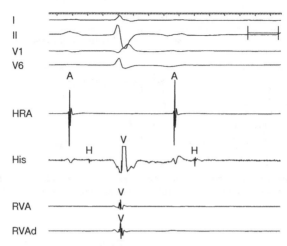

Figure 4.6 Electrograms from a patient with 2 : 1 AV block. In this case, the intracardiac electrograms show that the site of AV block is in infraHisian tissue.

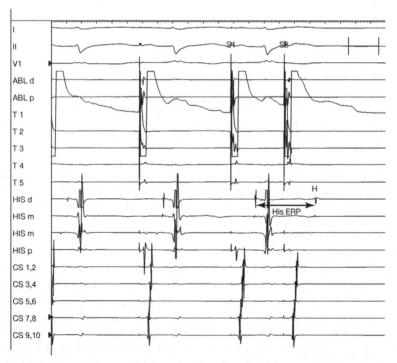

Figure 4.7 Atrial premature beat with a coupling interval of 350 ms leads to infraHisian block (His signal without a QRS). The HH interval is the His-Purkinje effective refractory period (His ERP).

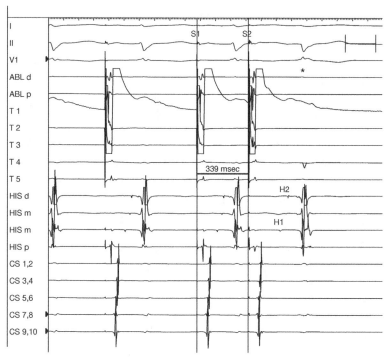

Figure 4.8 The atrial coupling interval is decreased to 340 ms. This leads to intraHisian delay and development of multiple His signals (H1 and H2). Delay within the His bundle allows recovery of infranodal tissue and a QRS complex is produced.

complex. Figure 3.4 (Chapter 3) shows an example of block within the AV node. In this case an atrial signal was not followed by a His signal.

AV refractoriness

Premature atrial extrastimuli provide important information on the relative refractory periods of different types of tissue on the atrioventricular conduction axis. Figures 4.7 to 4.10 illustrate this concept in a patient with intraHisian delay (the same patient as in Fig. 4.3). In Fig. 4.7, a premature atrial extrastimulus at a coupling interval of 350 ms results in infraHisian block. The His-Purkinje effective refractory period (ERP) can be calculated by the interval between the His signals. In Fig. 4.8, a slightly more premature atrial beat (coupling interval of 340 ms) results in intraHisian delay – notice the two components of the His signal (H1 and H2). This additional delay provides enough time so that the infraHisian tissue can conduct, and a ventricular electrogram (V) and a QRS complex are observed. The return of distal conduction due to the development of proximal conduction delay is called the "gap" phenomenon. In other words, delay in proximal tissue conduction allows the distal tissue to recover excitability and to be depolarized again. The gap phenomenon can occasionally be observed in all types of tissue. In Fig. 4.9, a more premature beat results

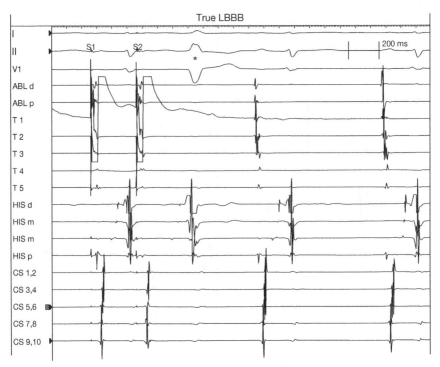

Figure 4.9 Shortening the coupling interval further to 290 ms results in greater AH delay and a change in the QRS morphology to a left bundle branch block pattern.

in a wide QRS complex with left bundle branch block (a predominantly negative QRS complex in V_1) because of the development of refractoriness in the left bundle. In Fig. 4.10, a slightly more premature atrial extrastimulus leads to a narrow QRS complex due to a longer HH interval due to AV nodal delay allowing both the right bundle and left bundle to recover and conduct normally. The gap phenomenon is not necessarily abnormal, and depends on the relative conduction and refractory properties of the different tissues that make up the atrioventricular conduction axis.

As a final word it must be acknowledged that, while important, at times electrophysiology evaluation for atrioventricular conduction is imperfect. Figure 4.11 shows the intracardiac electrograms from a patient with syncope and episodes of tachycardia noted on ambulatory ECG monitoring. Initial evaluation demonstrated an HV interval at the upper limits of normal (45 ms) with left bundle branch block. Atrial pacing protocols yielded no abnormalities and no evidence of infraHisian block. Fortuitously the patient suddenly developed infraHisian block with a very slow escape rate (< 30 beats per minute). A pacemaker was implanted and the patient has not had recurrent symptoms. As a corollary, although no catheter manipulation was being done when infraHisian block developed, this is an example of the electrophysiologic issues with placement of a pulmonary artery catheter in a patient with left

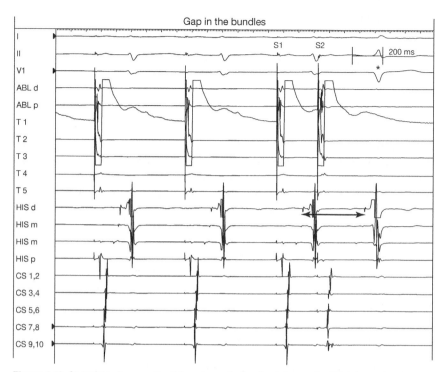

Figure 4.10 Shortening the coupling interval even further leads to greater AH delay and lengthening of the HH interval so both the right bundle branch and left bundle branch have recovered, resulting in a narrow QRS complex.

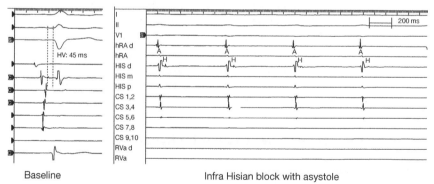

Figure 4.11 Intracardiac recordings from a patient with an episode of syncope. Baseline evaluation demonstrated left bundle branch block and a normal HV interval (45 ms). Atrial pacing protocols yielded no evidence of abnormal atrioventricular conduction. Fortuitously, near the end of the procedure the patient spontaneously developed high-grade infraHisian block.

bundle branch block. Slight mechanical trauma with pulmonary artery catheter placement can cause transient right bundle branch block, and in a patient with left bundle branch block (and dependent on right bundle conduction) this can lead to asystole.

CHAPTER 5

Supraventricular tachycardia

Electrophysiologic evaluation and ablation is frequently performed in patients with supraventricular tachycardia (SVT). In the last 20–25 years, ablation therapy has become an important treatment option that offers the potential for "cure" in some forms of supraventricular tachycardia. In the electrophysiology laboratory, the electrophysiologic mechanism and the anatomic substrate of supraventricular tachycardia can be studied by evaluating the methods of induction and termination, electrogram recording during tachycardia, responses to atrial and ventricular stimulation, and response to drugs. The reader should be warned that this chapter brings in a series of concepts that are sometimes difficult to keep straight. I can only say that with time the concepts will become second nature. Electrophysiologic properties for specific forms of supraventricular tachycardia are also discussed in Chapters 9 through 12, and reviewing this chapter after reading the chapters on specific arrhythmias may be very helpful.

Traditionally, tachycardias are classified by whether the QRS complex is wide or narrow. If a narrow QRS complex is present, the clinician knows that activation of the ventricles is occurring normally via the AV node and His–Purkinje system. Clinically, this classification scheme is *very* useful because some forms of wide complex tachycardias (ventricular tachycardia, ventricular fibrillation, and atrial fibrillation with activation of the ventricles via an accessory pathway) can be associated with significant hemodynamic compromise and death. However for "digging deeper" and understanding the electrophysiologic principles underlying supraventricular tachycardias, it is very helpful to also consider the classification of tachycardias by tissue/cellular mechanism and anatomic location.

Classification of supraventricular tachycardias

Cellular and tissue classification

On a cellular and tissue level, rapid heart rates can be due to three mechanisms: increased automaticity, triggered activity, and reentry (Fig. 5.1).

In automaticity, a cell or nest of cells displays spontaneous depolarization that leads to repetitive activation of Na^+ channels and rapid activity that can

Understanding Intracardiac EGMs and ECGs. By Fred Kusumoto. Published 2010 by Blackwell Publishing. ISBN: 978-1-4051-8410-6

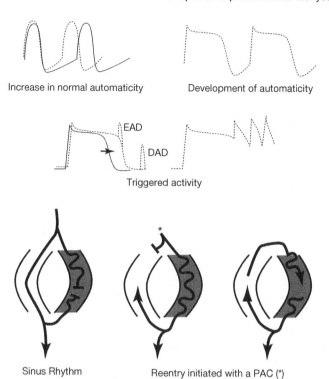

Increase in normal automaticity   Development of automaticity

Triggered activity

Sinus Rhythm   Reentry initiated with a PAC (*)

Figure 5.1 Cellular/tissue mechanisms for tachycardia. *Top row:* Increased automaticity can lead to faster heart rates. The most common example of this would be sinus tachycardia. Another possibility is development of automaticity in tissue that normally does not have pacemaker activity. *Middle row:* Triggered activity is a form of abnormal automaticity in which afterdepolarizations due to Na^+ and Ca^{2+} channel activation occur either during phase 3 (early afterdepolarizations, EAD) or after repolarization has completed (delayed afterdepolarizations, DAD). *Bottom row:* In reentry, two parallel paths with different conducting and refractory properties are present (slow pathway with shorter refractory periods in gray). During sinus rhythm the wave of depolarization conducts over the fast pathway and the depolarization wave is extinguished within the slow pathway. A premature beat (premature atrial contraction, PAC) can block in one pathway and conduct slowly down the second pathway. The wave of depolarization can enter the first pathway retrogradely, and if it does not encounter refractory tissue a self-perpetuating circuit can develop. (Reprinted with permission from Kusumoto FM. *ECG Interpretation: From Pathophysiology to Clinical Application*. New York, NY: Springer, 2009.)

propagate to the rest of the heart. The most common form of tachycardia due to increased automaticity is sinus tachycardia, where in response to sympathetic activation the sinus node depolarizes more rapidly, leading to a more rapid atrial and ventricular rate (if atrioventricular conduction is normal). Abnormal automaticity can be caused by rapid nonphysiologic activity from normal "pacemaker" cells in the heart such as the sinus node or AV node, or from development of automaticity in cells that normally do not demonstrate this property (ventricular or atrial myocytes).

Triggered activity is a special form of abnormal automaticity where prolongation of the action potential or increased intracellular Ca^{2+} leads to abnormal repetitive depolarizations. Both triggered activity and increased automaticity can be compared to repetitive drops into a still pond, with radial activation spreading outward like the circular ripples.

In reentry, two parallel paths with different electrophysiologic properties lead to the development of a continuous circuit analogous to "a dog chasing its tail" (Fig. 5.1). In reentry, a premature beat blocks in one of the pathways and conducts slowly down the parallel pathway, the wave of depolarization reenters the previously blocked pathway from the opposite direction, and a reentrant circuit can be formed. Although the process of reentry appears complicated and unlikely to occur, it is actually the most common cause of rapid heart rates.

In the electrophysiology laboratory it is important to distinguish between a tachycardia due to a "point source" from a cell or nest of cells that display abnormal automaticity and triggered activity or a "channel" that leads to reentry. Understanding the cellular mechanism helps the clinician design the appropriate method for ablating the arrhythmia.

Anatomic classification

Regardless of mechanism, it is also helpful to consider the anatomic location of the site that the tachycardia is emanating from (Fig. 5.2). There are essentially four anatomic sites within the heart that tachycardias can originate from: atrial tissue, the atrioventricular junctional area, ventricular tissue, or accessory pathways (often associated with arrhythmias that use the atria, the junction, the ventricles, and the accessory pathway). In supraventricular tachycardias, the ventricles are activated normally via the His–Purkinje system resulting in a narrow QRS complex. Since ventricular tachycardias and some accessory pathway-mediated tachycardias are associated with a wide complex tachycardia, for supraventricular tachycardias the clinician only has to consider tachycardias arising from atrial tissue or junctional tissue and one type of tachycardia associated with accessory pathways (Fig. 5.2).

In atrial tachycardias, the automatic site(s) or reentrant circuit is located within atrial tissue. An easy way to think of this is that if the ventricles and AV node region were separated from the atria, the tachycardia would continue. A stable reentrant circuit within the atria is traditionally called *atrial flutter*, while a point source of abnormal automaticity is called *focal atrial tachycardia*. A tachycardia due to several foci firing rapidly within the atria is called *multifocal atrial tachycardia*, and chaotic irregular activation of the atria is called *atrial fibrillation*.

Tachycardias from junctional tissue can be due to reentry or automaticity. The most common cause of regular supraventricular tachycardia in young adults is development of reentry within the AV node and adjacent atrial tissue. Logically, this type of supraventricular tachycardia is called *AV node reentry*. Abnormal automaticity from junctional tissue is less commonly observed and is usually called *junctional ectopic tachycardia*.

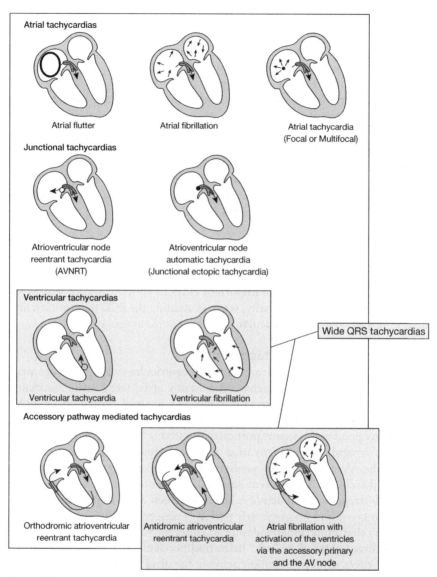

Figure 5.2 Anatomic tachycardia classification. Tachycardias can arise from atrial tissue, junctional tissue, ventricular tissue, or can utilize an accessory pathway. Tachycardias that arise from ventricular tissue, and some tachycardias associated with accessory pathways, produce wide QRS complex tachycardias and do not need to be considered in this discussion on supraventricular tachycardias. (Adapted with permission from Kusumoto FM. *Cardiovascular Pathophysiology*. Raleigh, NC: Hayes Barton Press, 1999.)

The final anatomic type of supraventricular tachycardia is due to the presence of an accessory pathway. Tachycardias due to accessory pathways and techniques for ablation will be covered in detail in Chapter 9. However, it is important to note that the presence of an accessory pathway connecting atrial and ventricular tissue is the classic example for the possible initiation of reentry, since the accessory pathway and the AV node form parallel pathways that connect atrial and ventricular tissue. Accessory pathways can be associated with supraventricular tachycardia if a reentrant circuit develops that activates the ventricles (anterograde conduction) via the AV node and activates the atria (retrograde conduction) via the accessory pathway. This type of supraventricular tachycardia is often called *atrioventricular (AV) reentry* to emphasize that both atrial and ventricular tissue are part of the reentrant circuit. Another term that is commonly added to describe this particular supraventricular tachycardia is *orthodromic AV reentry*. "Orthodromic" refers to normal conduction (*ortho* means straight/correct in Greek) over the AV node and normal depolarization of the ventricles. Unfortunately, having multiple names for the same tachycardia adds to the confusion for the newcomer to electrophysiology.

ECG in supraventricular tachycardia

The 12-lead ECG can provide important clues as to the cause of supraventricular tachycardia. Traditionally, when evaluating the ECG the clinician first determines whether the ventricular rate is regular or irregular.

Irregular supraventricular tachycardia

The most common causes for irregular supraventricular tachycardias are atrial fibrillation, multifocal atrial tachycardia, or any atrial tachycardia associated with an irregular ventricular response (Fig. 5.3). In atrial fibrillation, irregular continuous atrial activation leads to an ECG with no discrete isoelectric period. Since at any point in time some portion of the atria is depolarizing, the baseline is erratic. Irregular atrial activation leads to irregular impulses traveling through the AV node, and the ventricular rhythm is also irregular. In multifocal atrial tachycardia, different sites within the atria fire at different rates, leading to irregular atrial activity, but in between atrial depolarizations the atria are relaxed and an isoelectric period is observed. Think about three or four lights that blink independently at different rates. There will be times when all three lights will be "off." In the traditional model for atrial fibrillation, multiple waves of depolarization activate the atria continuously; perhaps a helpful analogy would be a white-water river, where continual waves of water crash from different directions, leading to constant activity.

A final cause for an irregular supraventricular tachycardias is a regular atrial tachycardia associated with irregular ventricular activation (Fig. 5.4). In this case atrial activity will display a rapid repetitive pattern that can usually be seen under the superimposed irregular QRS complexes and T waves due to ventricular depolarization and repolarization.

The astute reader will note that all of the causes for irregular supraventricular tachycardias are "atrial tachycardias." The irregular ventricular rate in atrial fibrillation and multifocal atrial tachycardia is due to irregular atrial

Atrial fibrillation

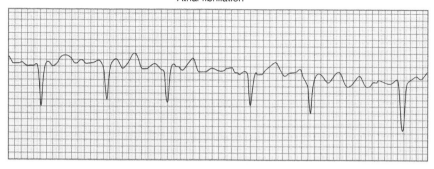

Multifocal atrial tachycardia

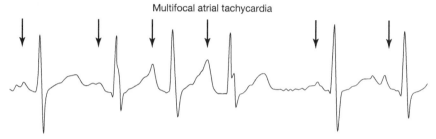

Figure 5.3 ECG examples of irregular tachycardias. In atrial fibrillation continuous fibrillatory activity will be observed, while in multifocal atrial tachycardia discrete P waves (arrows) with intervening isoelectric periods will be observed. (Reprinted with permission from Nicoll D, McPhee S, Pignone M, Lu CM, eds. *Pocket Guide to Diagnostic Tests*, 5th edn. New York, NY: McGraw-Hill, 2008).

activity, and the irregular ventricular rhythm in atrial tachycardia is due to varying conduction through the AV node.

Regular supraventricular tachycardia

Regular supraventricular tachycardias can be caused by rapid regular atrial tachycardias (due either to atrial flutter or to focal atrial tachycardia), tachycardias from the AV node region (reentry or, much more rarely, increased automaticity), or reentry using an accessory pathway.

When evaluating the ECG of a regular supraventricular tachycardia it is important to determine the location and the shape of the P wave (Fig. 5.5). In patients with tachycardia arising from the junctional area within or near the AV node, the atria and the ventricles are often depolarized simultaneously, and the P wave will usually be difficult to find because it is obscured by the QRS complex. In patients with atrioventricular reentry due to an accessory pathway the atria and ventricles are activated sequentially and the P wave will be observed after the QRS complex, usually within the ST segment. In patients with atrial tachycardia the location of the P wave relative to the QRS complex will depend on AV node conduction, so the location of the P wave

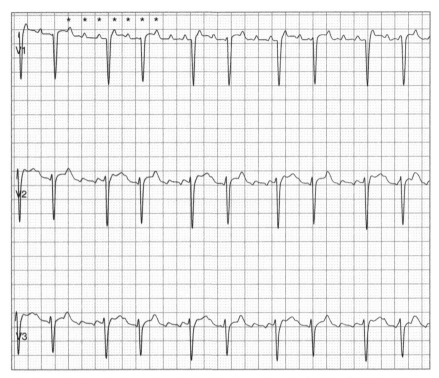

Figure 5.4 Atrial flutter with irregular ventricular response. Regular activation of the atria can be observed (*). However, because of varying AV nodal conduction the QRS complexes have an irregular rhythm. Notice, however, that there is a pattern to the irregular rhythm ("regularly irregular").

will vary depending on the atrial tachycardia rate and the AV node conduction properties of the patient. Generally, in atrial tachycardia the P wave will be observed before the QRS complex. Since the P wave is usually rather small compared to the QRS complex and the T wave, determining the site of the P wave can be difficult whatever the tachycardia type. One useful technique is to evaluate the QRS complex and T wave during both tachycardia and sinus rhythm. Any deflections that are observed during tachycardia that are not present during sinus rhythm probably represent P waves. In Fig. 5.6, deflections in the ST segment can be observed that are not present in sinus rhythm. This P wave location is most consistent with AV reentry using an accessory pathway.

Once P waves are identified, their morphology should be examined. Since the P waves are usually very small it is often difficult to distinguish subtle shape changes, but it is useful to decide whether the P waves are generally positive or negative in the inferior leads (II, III, and aVF). If the P waves are positive in these leads, it suggests that atrial activation is proceeding in a "high–low" direction, with depolarization toward the inferior leads. "High–low" atrial

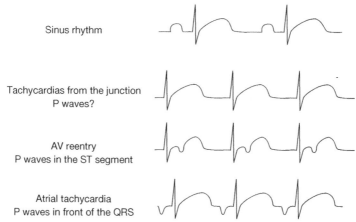

Figure 5.5 Usual location of P waves dependent on arrhythmia type. In arrhythmias arising from the junction, P waves will often be hard to see because they are obscured by the larger QRS complex. In AV reentry, sequential activation of the ventricles and the atria lead to P waves that can be more easily observed. Since retrograde conduction via the accessory pathway is usually faster than anterograde conduction over the AV node, the P wave is usually seen in the ST segment. In atrial tachycardias, the P wave will usually be seen before the QRS complex. These are general guidelines with many exceptions. For example, the relative positions of the P wave and QRS complex in an atrial tachycardia depends solely on a patient's atrioventricular conduction properties relative to the atrial tachycardia rate.

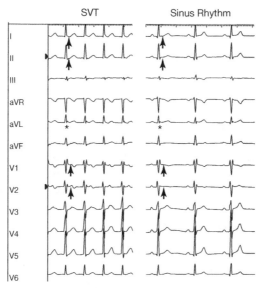

Figure 5.6 Comparison of sinus rhythm and supraventricular tachycardia (SVT) can be very useful. Deflections observed during SVT that are not seen during sinus rhythm (arrows) probably represent P waves during SVT. Conversely, deflections in the QRS or T waves that are seen during both sinus rhythm and SVT (*) represent ventricular depolarization or repolarization.

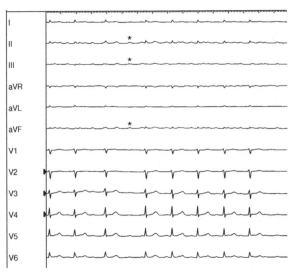

Figure 5.7 A patient with an atrial tachycardia arising from the superior vena cava–right atrial junction which leads to "high–low" atrial depolarization and positive P waves in the inferior leads.

activation is much more consistent with an atrial tachycardia and will not be seen if the atria are being activated retrogradely from the AV nodal region. Conversely, if the P waves are negative in the inferior leads it suggests that atrial activation is in the "low–high" direction, due either to retrograde activation via the AV node or accessory pathway or to a low atrial tachycardia focus. In Fig. 5.7, the P waves are positive in the inferior leads and negative in aVR. This patient has a focal atrial tachycardia arising from the superior vena cava–right atrial junction near the sinus node. Delay and intermittent block in the AV node causes the QRS complexes to be irregular. It is always easiest to evaluate the P wave morphology during pauses between the QRS complexes if possible. This allows evaluation of the P wave without interference from superimposed QRS complexes or T waves. Unfortunately, oftentimes it is difficult even to determine whether the P waves are positive or negative in the inferior leads. Reexamine Fig. 5.6. Although the P wave appears to be negative in lead II, it is certainly difficult to be truly confident of P wave morphology.

Electrophysiologic evaluation

Electrophysiologic testing provides the most comprehensive evaluation for patients with supraventricular tachycardia and provides special insight into the patterns observed on a surface ECG. Evaluating how tachycardias are initiated and terminate is useful for determining the mechanism. In addition, the ability to pace cardiac tissue – either the ventricles or the atria – during the tachycardia helps the clinician determine what tissues are required within the

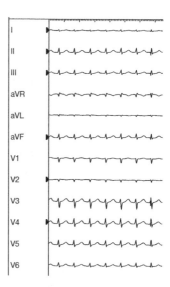

Figure 5.8 A 12-lead ECG obtained from a patient with supraventricular tachycardia. P waves cannot be seen.

tachycardia circuit and the underlying cellular/tissue mechanism responsible for the arrhythmia.

EGMs during tachycardia

The beauty of electrograms is that they take the "guesswork" out of trying to decide the location and shape of the P wave. Examine Fig. 5.8. This is a 12-lead ECG of a patient with a regular tachycardia. It is almost impossible to determine whether P waves are present, let alone to analyze their morphology. Now examine Fig. 5.9. Catheters are positioned within the ventricle, atria, coronary sinus, and His bundle region. The presence of intracardiac electrograms provides unequivocal evidence for the location of the P wave. In patients with atrial fibrillation, rapid irregular signals will be observed (Fig. 5.10). Although atrial fibrillation has become of greater interest to electrophysiologists over the last five years, and will be covered separately in Chapter 13, for the remainder of this discussion we will focus on using electrophysiologic testing for evaluating supraventricular tachycardias associated with regular atrial depolarization.

In fact, for practical purposes the great majority of regular supraventricular tachycardias will be due to one of three possibilities: (1) atrial tachycardia due to a focal source (focal atrial tachycardia) or reentry (atrial flutter), (2) AV node reentry, or (3) accessory pathway-mediated supraventricular tachycardia. The following discussion provides some of the basics for differentiating among these alternatives during electrophysiologic testing. Although this discussion may at times be difficult, and can seem incredibly complex to the newcomer to electrophysiology, it is worth emphasizing that in the end the clinician really just has to make a one-in-three choice.

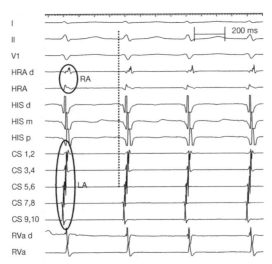

Figure 5.9 Intracardiac electrograms from the patient in Fig. 5.8. It can now be seen that the atria are being activated (ellipses showing left atrial (LA) and right atrial (RA) depolarization) at the same time as the QRS complex and are completely obscured by the QRS complex. As shown by the dotted line, atrial and ventricular depolarization are almost simultaneous. HRA, high right atrium; His, His bundle; CS, coronary sinus; RVa, right ventricular apex.

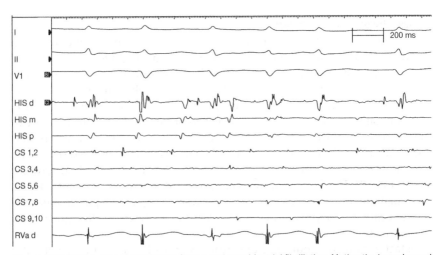

Figure 5.10 Intracardiac electrograms from a patient with atrial fibrillation. Notice the irregular and random atrial activation pattern observed in the coronary sinus electrograms.

Activation pattern of atrial depolarization

The pattern of atrial activation can be easily analyzed from intracardiac electrograms and provides the foundation for electrophysiology evaluation of supraventricular tachycardia. Analysis of the electrograms can provide clues for the general location of initial atrial activation: left atrium, right atrium, or septum. This can be done by looking at the relationship of atrial signals from electrodes located near the septum (most commonly a catheter placed superiorly near the His bundle straddling the right atrium and right ventricle, and the proximal electrodes from a catheter placed in the coronary sinus), the lateral left atrium (distal electrodes of the coronary sinus catheter), and the lateral right atrium (catheter placed near the superior vena cava and right atrial junction).

Examine the electrograms from three patients with supraventricular tachycardias in Fig. 5.11. Atrial electrograms can be identified by catheter and by timing: anything not occurring at the time of the QRS must be due to atrial activity, and any sharp large-amplitude electrogram recorded by a bipolar electrode pair placed within the atria must be due to atrial activity. In the top left panel, earliest atrial activation is in the right atrium. This pattern of atrial activation could be due to an atrial tachycardia arising from the right atrium or a right-sided accessory pathway leading to initial activation of the right atrium. Since the AV node is anatomically located in the septal region of the atria, it cannot be due to retrograde activation from the AV node. Similarly, in the bottom panel, earliest activation is in the distal coronary sinus catheter. This atrial activation pattern is most likely due to a left-sided accessory pathway or an atrial tachycardia from the left atrium. In the top right panel, earliest activation is in the His catheter recording. Here there are three possibilities, a septal accessory pathway, an atrial tachycardia located in the interatrial septum, or a tachycardia arising from the AV node with retrograde atrial activation. Activation of the atria from a site away from the septal area is often collectively called "eccentric activation" to emphasize that retrograde AV nodal conduction is much less likely. In this figure the patient in the left panel has a right atrial tachycardia and the patients in the top right and bottom panels have septal and left-sided accessory pathways respectively. It is impossible to make a specific diagnosis in any of the three cases solely from analyzing the atrial activation pattern, although, as just mentioned, AV node reentry is unlikely in the presence of eccentric atrial activation.

In addition to deciding "which side" of the atria is activated earliest, it is also useful to determine whether atrial activation is "high–low" or "low–high" and whether atrial activity appears to arise from the AV nodal region. Patients with earliest atrial activity in the superior portion of the right or left atrium make retrograde activation via the AV node or an accessory pathway unlikely. Activation from the AV node region will have earliest atrial signals in catheters located near the atrial septum, usually the proximal electrodes of a catheter placed in the coronary sinus or a catheter placed at the His bundle region. In the top panel of Fig. 5.11, the first atrial electrogram is observed in a catheter placed in the high right atrium at the superior vena cava–right atrial junction, confirming a "high–low" atrial activation pattern and suggests the presence of an atrial tachycardia.

Another important point is to consider whether or not electrical signals can be recorded throughout the cycle length. In patients with atrial flutter due to

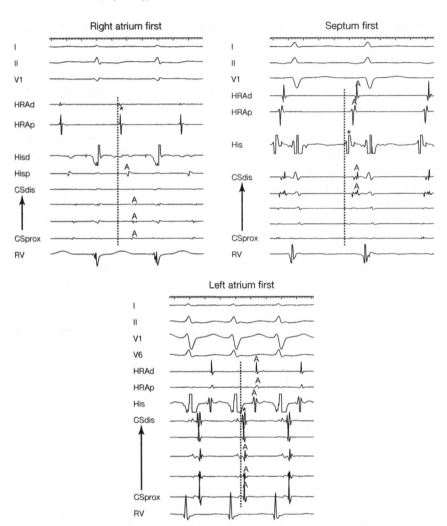

Figure 5.11 Supraventricular tachycardias (notice the narrow QRS complex) from three patients. In all three examples the earliest site of atrial activation is designated by a dotted line and asterisk. *Top left:* Earliest atrial activation occurs in the right atrium. *Top right:* earliest atrial activation occurs in the His catheter. *Bottom:* Earliest atrial activation is in the distal coronary sinus. A, atrial electrograms.

a large macroreentrant circuit, atrial electrograms can often be recorded through-out the tachycardia cycle. In Fig. 5.12, electrograms from a patient with a focal atrial tachycardia and a patient with atrial flutter are shown. The T electro-grams are recorded from a decapolar catheter that is placed along the tricuspid annulus (fluoroscopy of the catheter position is shown in Fig. 12.3, Chapter 12 – but the location of the catheter is really unimportant for our discussion here). In the top panel, the electrograms from a patient with atrial flutter span the

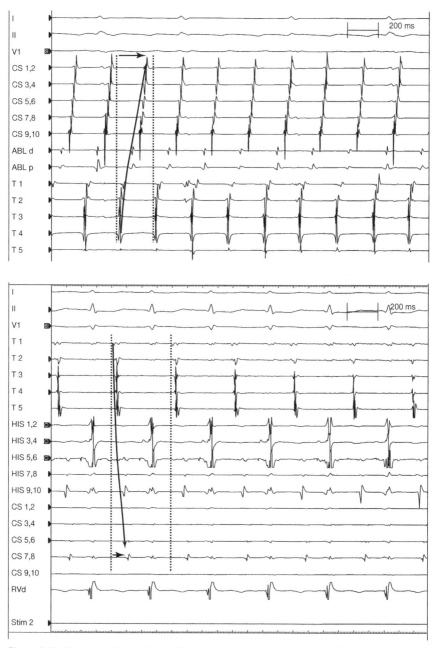

Figure 5.12 *Top:* In a patient with atrial flutter due to a large macroreentrant circuit, the tachycardia cycle length (dotted lines) will sometimes be completely spanned by electrograms. *Bottom:* In a patient with a focal atrial tachycardia, between each atrial depolarization there is a quiescent period. The atria are activated rapidly from the "point source."

entire tachycardia cycle length. In contrast, in a patient with a focal atrial tachycardia, electrograms are recorded during only 25% of the tachycardia cycle. Although both focal atrial tachycardia and atrial flutter can be considered "atrial tachycardias" in a general sense, they have very different mechanisms. A focal atrial tachycardia can be compared to a "blinking light" while atrial flutter is like a "dog chasing its tail." Simultaneous atrial activation of disparate chambers is not the only characteristic of focal atrial tachycardia. Rapid atrial activation taking up only a small portion of the tachycardia cycle length can also be seen if the tachycardia has periods where signals are not measured within the atria. For example, since temporally a large portion of the reentrant wave of depolarization in AV node reentry is spent within the AV node, atrial activity will occur simultaneously. Similarly in orthodromic AV reentrant tachycardia, atrial activation makes up only one component of the tachycardia circuit. The other portions of the tachycardia circuit involve the AV node and His bundle, ventricular tissue, and conduction over the accessory pathway. Reexamining the middle and right panels of Fig. 5.11, one can see that atrial activation takes up only a small portion of the tachycardia cycle length. The "take-home message" is that in most cases, if atrial electrograms can be recorded by catheters throughout the entire tachycardia cycle length, atrial flutter is the most likely diagnosis/mechanism. On the other hand, if atrial electrograms can be recorded in only a small portion of the cycle length, an atrial flutter could still be present (catheters cannot be simultaneously placed in all portions of the atria) or any of the other mechanisms/types of supraventricular tachycardia could be present.

Temporal relationship of atrial and ventricular activation

If the tachycardia continues even in the setting of 2 : 1 atrial–ventricular relationship it rules out AV reentrant tachycardia, which must use ventricular tissue as a necessary part of the circuit. In the top panel of Fig. 5.12, there are two atrial electrograms for every QRS complex.

Another useful finding for ruling out accessory pathway-mediated tachycardia is the presence of simultaneous atrial and ventricular activity, since a certain amount of time is required during sequential ventricular and atrial activation. Reexamine the electrograms in Fig. 5.9. Notice that the atrial electrograms are occurring at the same time as the QRS complex. In a supraventricular tachycardia utilizing an accessory pathway, after ventricular activation via the His–Purkinje system a finite amount of time is required for the wave of depolarization to travel through ventricular tissue, travel over the accessory pathway, and retrogradely activate the atria. Josephson and colleagues suggest that a VA interval < 65 ms rules out an accessory pathway. When simultaneous atrial and ventricular depolarization is observed (VA interval of 0 ms) as in Fig. 5.9, a tachycardia arising from the junctional region is most likely, although an atrial tachycardia with significant first-degree AV block is still possible.

Initiation and spontaneous termination

If the tachycardia terminates spontaneously with an atrial electrogram it makes atrial tachycardia very unlikely, since it implies that the AV node is an essential part of the circuit. In an atrial tachycardia, the tachycardia "does not care" whether AV node conduction is present, so if an atrial tachycardia terminates the last atrial impulse will generally lead to a ventricular beat. An example of this is shown in Figs. 5.13 and 5.14. Figure 5.13 shows a patient with a supraventricular tachycardia with earliest atrial activation in the distal coronary sinus. Given eccentric atrial activation the two possibilities are a left-sided accessory pathway or a focal atrial tachycardia from the left atrium. The tachycardia spontaneously terminates on an atrial electrogram and, as shown in Fig. 5.14, this effectively rules out atrial tachycardia and confirms the diagnosis of a left-sided accessory pathway in this patient. Unfortunately termination of a supraventricular tachycardia with a ventricular electrogram provides no information on the mechanism of the tachycardia since atrial tachycardia, AV node reentry, and orthodromic AV reentry can all terminate with ventricular depolarization: the atrial tachycardia simply stops and ventricular depolarization follows; AV node reentry terminates and the last reentrant cycle yields a QRS complex; orthodromic AV reentry terminates due to retrograde block in the accessory pathway.

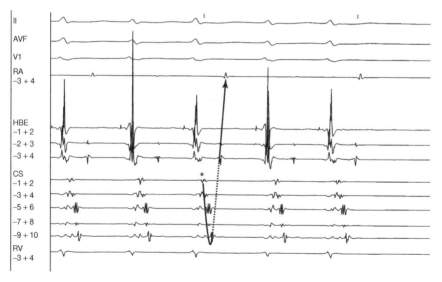

Figure 5.13 A patient with supraventricular tachycardia with earliest atrial activation at the distal coronary sinus (*). Atrial depolarization travels sequentially from distal to proximal in the coronary sinus electrograms, His bundle, and finally the high right atrium. This atrial activation pattern could be observed in a patient with a left-sided accessory pathway or a focal atrial tachycardia from the left atrium. However, the tachycardia spontaneously terminates on an atrial electrogram, ruling out atrial tachycardia (see Fig. 5.14).

AV reentry
If the reentrant circuit
terminates due to development
of block in the AV node, the last
electrogram will be due to atrial activation

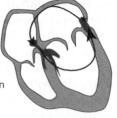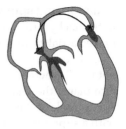

Atrial tachycardia
With termination, the last
beat of atrial tachycardia will
lead to a QRS

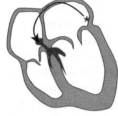

Figure 5.14 Schematic of spontaneous termination of supraventricular tachycardia due to a left-sided accessory pathway or a focal atrial tachycardia. If a focal atrial tachycardia "stops," the last atrial depolarization will lead to a QRS complex since the ventricular activation is following passively via atrioventricular conduction.

Response to stimuli

Ventricular premature beats

Delivery of premature ventricular beats is the mainstay of programmed stimulation during supraventricular tachycardia. Remember that supraventricular tachycardia can be due to tachycardia mechanisms in the atria, or within or near the AV node, or can utilize an accessory pathway. Ventricular stimulation will have varying likelihood of interacting with different types of tachycardias. In a patient with an accessory pathway the tachycardia circuit is quite large, so it is easy to interact with the circuit. Ventricular stimuli are least likely to interact with atrial tachycardia, since the ventricular stimulus must conduct through ventricular tissue, the right bundle, the His bundle, the AV node, and any intervening atrial tissue before it can potentially interact with the tachycardia site.

Several responses to ventricular stimulation are useful for differentiating between atrial tachycardia, AV node reentry, and accessory pathway-mediated supraventricular tachycardia. Using the technique described in Chapter 3 and illustrated in Figs. 3.22 to 3.24, the clinician will set up the cardiac stimulator to sense intrinsic signals during the tachycardia and deliver a single ventricular extrastimulus at specific intervals after the last sensed beat. First, a ventricular extrastimulus is delivered at the time of His bundle depolarization ("V on His"). If a ventricular stimulus delivered at the time the His bundle is refractory resets the tachycardia, an alternative route of atrial activation other than

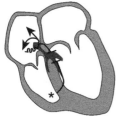
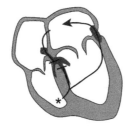
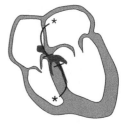

AV node reentry	AV reentry	Atrial tachycardia
PVC cannot interact with the tachycardia	PVC leads to early atrial activation	PVC cannot interact with the tachycardia

Figure 5.15 Schematic showing the importance of evaluating a "V on His" response (specifically placed premature ventricular contraction, PVC). In patients with atrial tachycardia or AV node reentry, a V on His will not affect the tachycardia because the His bundle is refractory. On the other hand, if a V on His resets the tachycardia with the same atrial activation sequence it confirms the presence of an accessory pathway that is participating in the supraventricular tachycardia (atrioventricular reentry).

the AV node/His bundle must be present (Fig. 5.15). If the atrial activation pattern is unaltered, resetting the tachycardia can only occur if an accessory pathway-mediated supraventricular tachycardia is present.

Figure 5.16 shows the electrograms from a patient with a supraventricular tachycardia. The earliest discernible atrial signal appears to be in the high right atrial catheter (*), although an atrial signal obscured by the ventricular electrogram may be present in the His bundle. A ventricular stimulus (S_2) delivered

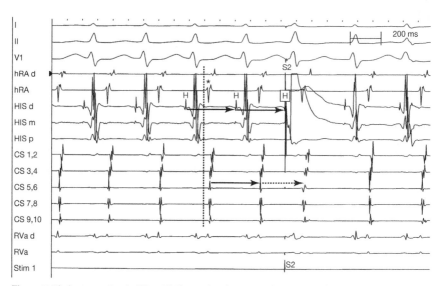

Figure 5.16 An example of a "V on His" resetting the tachycardia in a patient with an accessory pathway. A ventricular extrastimulus (S_2) delivered when the His bundle has already depolarized (H) leads to early atrial activation (resets the tachycardia).

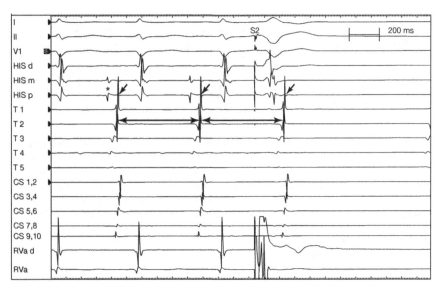

Figure 5.17 A very premature ventricular extrastimulus (S_2) terminates the tachycardia without resetting atrial depolarization. This response rules out atrial tachycardia. The ten electrode catheter labeled T is located in the lateral wall of the right atrium.

near the His bundle is delivered (notice the slight change in the QRS complex) at the same time that the His bundle depolarizes; a His bundle signal (H) can be seen just before the ventricular stimulus. Notice that the S_2 causes earlier atrial depolarization (dotted arrow), confirming the presence of an accessory pathway.

In addition to delivering a ventricular extrastimulus at the time of His bundle depolarization, responses to earlier ventricular depolarizations can also be useful. Figure 5.17 shows a patient with a supraventricular tachycardia with earliest atrial activation in the His bundle region (*). This activation pattern could be due to focal atrial tachycardia from the interatrial septum, AV node reentry with slow retrograde activation of the atria (this form of AV node reentry is called "atypical" and will be discussed more fully in Chapter 10), or an accessory pathway with slow conduction properties. If one simply uses "usual" P wave location for different tachycardia types (Fig. 5.5), atrial tachy-cardia would be the most likely diagnosis. A very premature ventricular extrastimulus (S_2) is delivered that leads to termination of the tachycardia without affecting the tachycardia cycle length (double-headed arrows). This response is called "termination without reset." The only way a premature ven-tricular extrastimulus can terminate an atrial tachycardia is if the premature ventricular stimulus leads to premature atrial depolarization. The presence of "termination without reset" by a ventricular extrastimulus rules out atrial tachycardia, leaving AV node reentry or an accessory pathway-mediated tachycardia as the only possibilities. The astute reader will notice that a low-amplitude low-frequency signal that may represent His bundle activation can

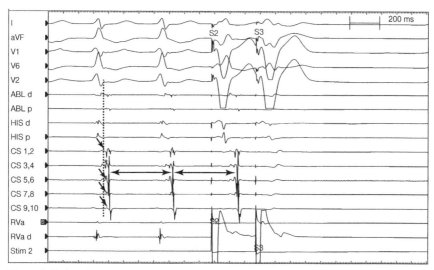

Figure 5.18 A patient with a supraventricular tachycardia with earliest atrial activation in the coronary sinus (*). Two ventricular extrastimuli (S_2 and S_3) lead to termination of the tachycardia without resetting atrial depolarization and without an atrial depolarization after the second premature ventricular stimulus. See text for details.

be seen (small diagonal arrows), and that these also are not reset by the ventricular extrastimulus. If one believes that these signals represent His bundle depolarizations this response would also rule out AV node reentry, leaving a slowly conducting accessory pathway as the only tenable diagnosis. It is difficult to make definitive decisions with such small signals (which may represent artifact from far-field activation), but several other responses did confirm that this patient had a slowly conducting accessory pathway as the cause of his supraventricular tachycardia.

Figure 5.18 shows another example of ventricular extrastimuli terminating a supraventricular tachycardia. In this case the patient has a supraventricular tachycardia with earliest atrial activation at electrodes 3,4 of the coronary sinus catheter (*). In this example of eccentric atrial activation, a left-sided accessory pathway or a focal left atrial tachycardia is most likely. Two ventricular extrastimuli (S_2 and S_3) are delivered without resetting the interval between the atrial electrograms (double-headed arrows), and the S_3 is not associated with an accompanying atrial electrogram. This response to ventricular stimulation of "termination without an A" rules out atrial tachycardia. A schematic for this is shown in Fig. 5.19. If a premature ventricular stimulus blocks ventricular activation in the AV node (no accompanying atrial electrogram) then an atrial tachycardia will continue. Termination of the tachycardia without an atrial electrogram suggests that the AV node forms an essential part of the tachycardia circuit (AV node reentry or accessory pathway-mediated atrioventricular reentry).

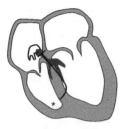
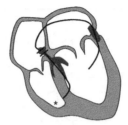
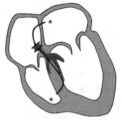

AV node reentry	AV reentry	Atrial tachycardia
PVC may terminate the tachycardia within the AV node	PVC may terminate the tachycardia within the AV node	PVC may be associated with AV block but the tachycardia will continue

Figure 5.19 Schematic showing responses of different tachycardia types to ventricular stimuli. Both AV node reentry and accessory pathway-mediated atrioventricular reentry can be terminated by a ventricular stimulus without an accompanying atrial depolarization because it produces refractory tissue within the AV node. However, although a premature ventricular stimulus can cause transient block in the AV node, the atrial tachycardia will not be affected and will continue.

In fact "AV node dependence" is one of the important ECG methods for classifying supraventricular tachycardias. An AV node-independent tachycardia will continue in the presence of AV node block, whereas an AV node dependent tachycardia will terminate with AV block. Electrophysiologic signs for the presence of an AV node dependent tachycardia include spontaneous termination on an atrial electrogram, and termination of the tachycardia with a ventricular extrastimulus without reset or an accompanying atrial signal. Atrial tachycardias are "AV node independent." Supraventricular tachycardias due to AV reentry are "AV node dependent." AV node reentry is almost always "AV node dependent," although sometimes continuation of the tachycardia in the presence of AV block can be seen, due to atrioventricular block "below" the site of AV node reentry (see Fig. 10.14, Chapter 10).

Atrial premature beats

Delivery of atrial stimuli during tachycardia provides far less information than ventricular stimuli, but it can be useful, particularly for helping determine the mechanism for a tachycardia. Figure 5.20 shows a 12-lead ECG from a patient with an irregular supraventricular tachycardia. No P waves can be seen on the 12-lead ECG. The electrograms from the patient are shown in Fig. 5.21. The atrial and ventricular electrograms are simultaneous, ruling out an accessory pathway-mediated AV reentry. In addition, despite the irregular QRS intervals the relationship between the ventricular and atrial signals remains constant. "Hooking" of ventricular and subsequent atrial depolarization despite changes in cycle length makes atrial tachycardia unlikely. Remember that there is no obligate fixed relationship between atrial and ventricular depolarization in atrial tachycardia (Fig. 5.22). The atrial tachycardia focus simply "fires" and does not care what the AV node conduction is. Another way to

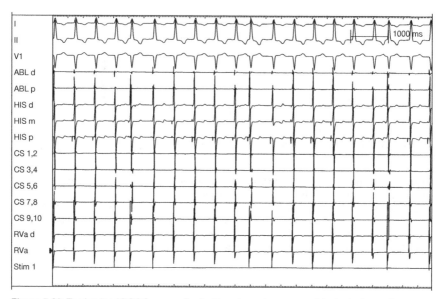

Figure 5.20 Twelve-lead ECG from a patient with an irregular supraventricular tachycardia. No P waves can be seen.

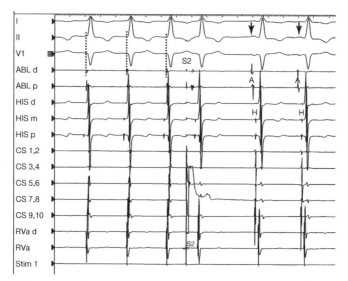

Figure 5.21 Electrograms from the patient in Fig. 5.20. Notice that the relationship between atrial depolarization and the QRS complexes (dotted lines) is fixed despite changes in the tachycardia cycle length. A premature atrial extrastimulus delivered from the coronary sinus catheter terminates the tachycardia (see text).

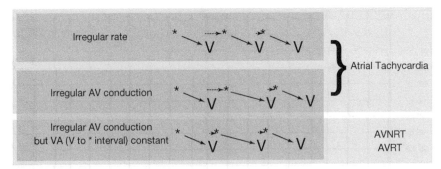

Figure 5.22 Irregular ventricular rates can be present in atrial tachycardia due to irregular rate of atrial depolarization (*) or changes in AV conduction due to varying refractoriness of the AV node. In either case the ventricular–atrial relationship will change since the atrial tachycardia is associated with the subsequent QRS, not the preceding QRS. The presence of a constant ventricular–atrial interval ("hooking") suggests that retrograde atrial activation is present. AVNET: AV node reentrant tachycardia; AVET: Atrioventricular reentrant tachycardia

think about this is that in an atrial tachycardia, atrial depolarization causes subsequent ventricular depolarization and there is no fixed relationship with the preceding QRS. In this case the patient could have AV node reentry that uses several different reentrant circuits or irregular depolarization from an automatic site within the AV node. Termination of the tachycardia with a premature atrial extrastimulus makes reentry much more likely.

Response to drugs

The most common drug response studied in the electrophysiology laboratory is the response to adenosine during tachycardia. Adenosine acts to block the AV node and will terminate tachycardias that are AV node dependent. Unfortunately adenosine will also terminate atrial tachycardias due to triggered activity. Adenosine is helpful if the tachycardia continues in the presence of AV nodal block since this finding essentially "rules in" the presence of an atrial tachycardia. In Fig. 5.23, a patient has a supraventricular tachycardia with earliest atrial activation in the lateral wall of the right atrium (T2). Eccentric atrial activation is present, with the right atrial electrogram occurring well before the interatrial septum (His 9,10) or the left atrium (CS) signals. In this case the patient has a focal right atrial tachycardia or a slowly conducting right-sided accessory pathway. The tachycardia continues even with atrioventricular block produced by adenosine infusion. This response "rules out" accessory pathway-mediated AV reentry (in which the AV node is an essential part of the tachycardia circuit) and establishes a diagnosis of focal right atrial tachycardia. The usual dose range for adenosine during electrophysiology studies is 3–6 mg, since the drug is usually given centrally through large sheaths.

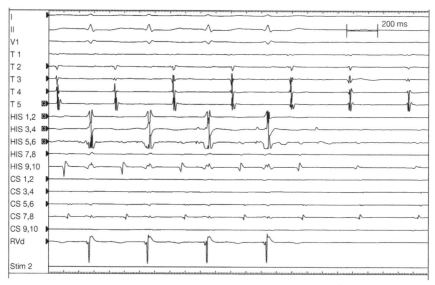

Figure 5.23 Response to adenosine. In this patient with supraventricular tachycardia, earliest atrial activation is noted in a ten-electrode catheter placed in the lateral wall of the right atrium near the tricuspid annulus (T1 through T5). In this case of eccentric atrial activation the two most likely possibilities are a right-sided accessory pathway or a focal right atrial tachycardia. With adenosine infusion-induced AV block the tachycardia continues, thus ruling out accessory pathway-mediated AV reentry and establishing a diagnosis of a focal right atrial tachycardia.

Summary

This chapter has necessarily described a dizzying array of concepts that can be difficult to integrate for the student just learning electrophysiology. However, evaluation of intracardiac electrograms in patients with supraventricular tachycardias remains the most important skill in clinical electrophysiology. Table 5.1 provides an overview of the process for evaluating atrial electrograms during an electrophysiology studies. Table 5.2 provides important information for distinguishing between the three types of regular tachycardia that are commonly observed during electrophysiology studies: atrial tachycardia, AV node reentry, and accessory pathway-mediated AV reentry. Finally, Fig. 5.24 provides the same information in a flowchart to provide the student a working process for evaluating a regular supraventricular tachycardia in the electrophysiology laboratory. Again, the reader is encouraged to return to this chapter after reading about the individual aspects of different types of supraventricular tachycardias.

Table 5.1 Evaluation of atrial electrograms during supraventricular tachycardia.

Question	Electrograms
Is organized atrial activity present?	If the atrial signals are very rapid and irregular, atrial fibrillation is present
What is the general atrial activation pattern?	If earliest atrial activity is from septal catheters/electrodes consider a tachycardia source near the AV junction
	If earliest atrial activity is in the right atrium consider a tachycardia focus within the right atrium or a right-sided accessory pathway
	If earliest atrial activity is in the coronary sinus, consider a left-sided atrial tachycardia or a left-sided accessory pathway
	A "high–low" activation pattern makes atrial tachycardia more likely
Are there more atrial signals than ventricular signals?	If so, atrial flutter or a focal atrial tachycardia is most likely
If atrial and ventricular tachycardia have a 1 : 1 relationship what is the temporal relationship between atrial and ventricular activity?	In tachycardias arising from the junctional region, simultaneous atrial and ventricular activity leads to a very short VA conduction
	In accessory pathway tachycardias sequential ventricular and atrial activation leads to atrial activity sometime after the QRS complex
	In atrial tachycardia atrial activity will be observed before ventricular activity

Table 5.2 Clues for distinguishing between different types of regular supraventricular tachycardia.

	EGMs during tachycardia	"Rules out"	"Rules in"
Atrial tachycardia	Atrial activity usually precedes ventricular activity but can be "anywhere" – with the specific location dependent on the atrial rate and AV node conduction properties	PVC terminates SVT without A PVC terminates SVT without reset Spontaneous termination with an A	
AV node reentry	Typically the atrial and ventricular signals will be simultaneous, but almost any relationship can be seen in atypical forms.	"High–low" atrial activation	
Accessory pathway-mediated AV reentry	Atrial activation will occur after ventricular activation	Simultaneous V and A signals A : V relationship is not 1 : 1 during tachycardia "High–low" atrial activation	PVC when the His is refractory resets SVT Cycle length of the tachycardia changes with the development of bundle branch block (discussed in Chapter 9)

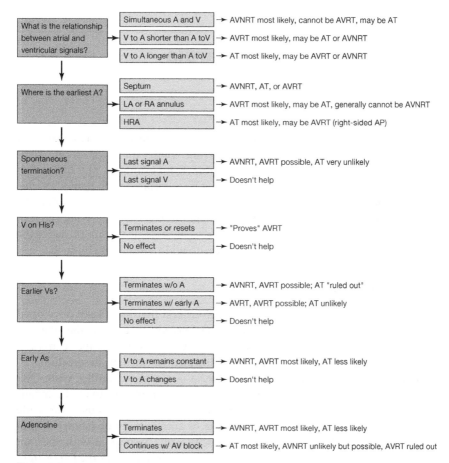

Figure 5.24 Flowchart for evaluation of regular supraventricular tachycardia in the electrophysiology laboratory.

CHAPTER 6

Wide complex tachycardia

Wide complex tachycardia can represent either ventricular tachycardia or supraventricular tachycardia with aberrant ventricular activation (right bundle branch block or left bundle branch block, for example). This distinction is critical, since ventricular tachycardia can be associated with hemodynamic compromise. Because of its availability and ease of use, the surface ECG is the standard and most clinically used tool for identifying the underlying cause of wide complex tachycardia. However, electrophysiologic testing provides the most definitive evaluation for the patient with wide complex tachycardia.

ECG evaluation

A comprehensive discussion on the many criteria that have been developed for analyzing an ECG in wide complex tachycardia is beyond the scope of a book focused on electrophysiology. However, it is instructive to discuss analysis of QRS morphology and identifying atrioventricular dissociation.

By definition a wide complex tachycardia is associated with a wide QRS complex > 0.12 seconds. The presence of a wide complex tachycardia means that ventricular activation is not normal. The two main causes for wide complex tachycardia are an abnormal site of automaticity or reentry within ventricular tissue or a supraventricular tachycardia associated with aberrant activation of the ventricles due to blocked conduction in either the left or right bundle or, more rarely, via an accessory pathway (Fig. 6.1). The morphology criteria try to distinguish characteristics associated with bundle branch block from those characteristics not associated with bundle branch block.

In right bundle branch block, the left ventricle is activated before the right ventricle. Late activation of the right ventricle leads to a positive QRS complex in V_1 and a QRS complex in V_6 with a late negative wave (Fig. 6.2). A broadly positive QRS complex in V_1 associated with a positive wide QRS complex in V_6 would be very atypical for right bundle branch block and makes ventricular tachycardia more likely. In fact the presence of positive concordance in the precordial leads (V_1–V_6) is an excellent clue for the presence of ventricular tachycardia.

In left bundle branch block, the right ventricle is activated before the left ventricle so the QRS complex in V_1 is negative and the QRS complex in V_6 is

Understanding Intracardiac EGMs and ECGs. By Fred Kusumoto. Published 2010 by Blackwell Publishing. ISBN: 978-1-4051-8410-6

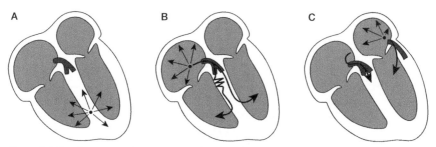

Figure 6.1 Possible causes for wide complex tachycardia. (*A*) A tachycardia site in ventricular tissue (automaticity or reentry). (*B*) Any supraventricular tachycardia associated with bundle branch block. (*C*) A supraventricular tachycardia associated with activation of the ventricles via an accessory pathway. (Reprinted with permission from Kusumoto FM. *Cardiovascular Pathophysiology*. Raleigh, NC: Hayes Barton Press, 1999.)

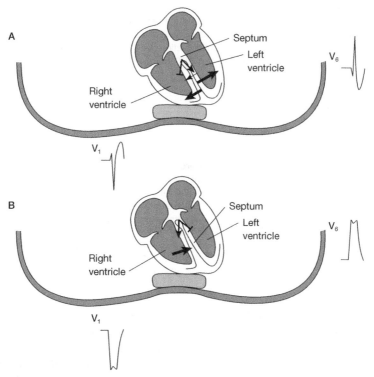

Figure 6.2 ECG in left and right bundle branch block. (*A*) In right bundle branch block left-to-right septal activation is normal, since the left bundle branch depolarizes normally. Depolarization of the left ventricle yields a right-to-left wave of activation. Finally the right ventricle is activated late from left to right. In V_1 an rSR′ complex is recorded and in V_6 a qRS complex is seen. (*B*) In left bundle branch block, right-to-left septal activation and late right-to-left activation of the left ventricle leads to a wide negative complex in V_1 and a wide positive complex in V_6. (Reprinted with permission from Kusumoto FM. *Cardiovascular Pathophysiology*. Raleigh, NC: Hayes Barton Press, 1999.)

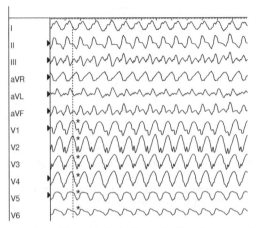

Figure 6.3 ECG from a patient with ventricular tachycardia. Negative concordance is present in the precordial leads, with all negative QRS complexes (*). This means that activation of the ventricles is occurring from the anterior apex of the left ventricle. Sometimes it can be difficult to determine where the QRS starts. Since the ECG is recorded simultaneously a vertical line can be drawn from the site of a QRS where the initial deflection can easily be seen (V_5 in this case), and this will serve as a marker that helps determine QRS morphology.

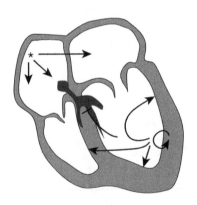

Figure 6.4 Schematic showing AV dissociation in ventricular tachycardia. A reentrant circuit develops at the site of the scar, and leads to repetitive abnormal depolarization of the ventricles. The sinus node is unaffected and continues to activate the atria (it does not "care" about ventricular activation). (Reprinted with permission from Kusumoto FM. *ECG Interpretation: From Pathophysiology to Clinical Application*. New York, NY: Springer, 2009.)

usually positive (Fig. 6.2). The presence of a negative QRS complex in both V_1 and V_6 would be unlikely to represent left bundle branch block and would more likely represent ventricular tachycardia. This is the reason that negative concordance, or negative QRS complexes in all of the precordial leads, is an excellent ECG criterion for ventricular tachycardia (Fig. 6.3). If all of the precordial QRS complexes are negative then depolarization must be initiated from the left ventricular apical region. This type of activation pattern would not be seen in left bundle branch block.

The presence of independent atrial and ventricular activity (AV dissociation) is diagnostic for ventricular tachycardia in most circumstances (Fig. 6.4). On the surface ECG, atrioventricular dissociation is most easily identified by

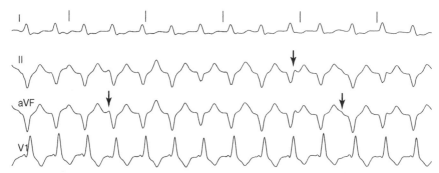

Figure 6.5 ECG showing AV dissociation. Notice the "unexpected" deflections that must represent atrial activity and AV dissociation (arrows). Evidence for atrial activity can be subtle; it is useful to scan the entire ECG for evidence of AV dissociation. (Reprinted with permission from Kusumoto FM. *ECG Interpretation: From Pathophysiology to Clinical Application*. New York, NY: Springer, 2009.)

finding "unexpected" deflections during the 12-lead ECG that must represent P waves that are not related to ventricular activation (Fig. 6.5). Remember that if a patient has a ventricular arrhythmia due to a focal or reentrant cause, in some cases retrograde conduction will be blocked. This is analogous to our discussion in Chapter 4 for determining the retrograde AV blocked cycle length. Unfortunately atrioventricular dissociation may be difficult to identify by the surface ECG. In addition, if the ventricular rate is slow enough, 1 : 1 ventriculoatrial conduction may be present.

Electrophysiologic evaluation

As in supraventricular tachycardia, electrophysiologic testing provides the best tool for evaluating a patient with wide complex tachycardia. Fortunately, analysis of wide complex tachycardia is easier to discuss in this introductory text, since the main clinical issue is to determine whether ventricular tachycardia is present.

Relationship between atrial and ventricular activity

Placing a catheter within the atrium provides unequivocal evidence for the timing of atrial activity. If atrial activity is independent of or intermittently associated with ventricular activity, atrioventricular dissociation is present and ventricular tachycardia overwhelmingly becomes the most likely diagnosis. The situation is analogous to continued atrial tachycardia in the presence of AV block making atrial tachycardia the most likely diagnosis in patients with supraventricular tachycardia. In Fig. 6.6, the 12-lead ECG from a patient with an irregular wide complex tachycardia is shown. Since the tachycardia had an irregular rhythm the patient was erroneously given the clinical diagnosis of atrial fibrillation – although there are several ECG clues suggesting that this was probably not the correct diagnosis, including the presence of positive

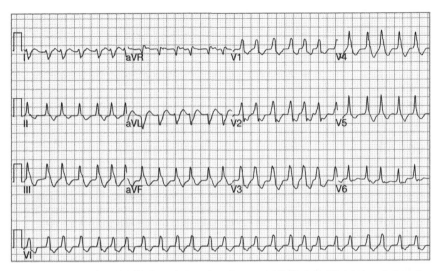

Figure 6.6 ECG from a patient who was thought to have atrial fibrillation with right bundle branch block. It would be very unusual for right bundle branch block to be associated with a positive QRS complex in V_6. (Reprinted with permission from Kusumoto FM. *ECG Interpretation: From Pathophysiology to Clinical Application.* New York, NY: Springer, 2009.)

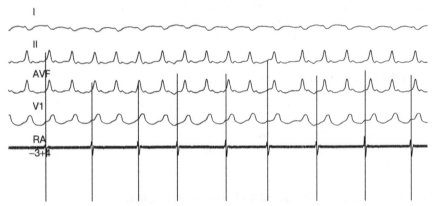

Figure 6.7 The patient from Fig. 6.6 had a quadripolar electrode catheter placed in the right atrium. Notice that atrial activity is organized (atrial fibrillation would have displayed rapid activity) and dissociated from ventricular activity, confirming the presence of ventricular tachycardia. (Reprinted with permission from Kusumoto FM. *ECG Interpretation: From Pathophysiology to Clinical Application.* New York, NY: Springer, 2009.)

concordance in the precordial leads. The patient was brought to the electro-physiology laboratory, where the diagnosis of ventricular tachycardia was confirmed by the presence of AV dissociation (Fig. 6.7).

There are two very rare conditions in which true AV dissociation can be observed in the setting of wide complex tachycardia. The first is a tachycardia

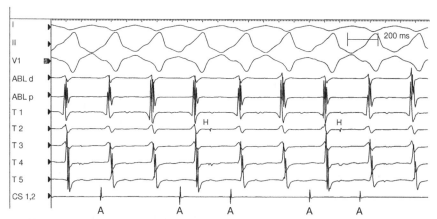

Figure 6.8 Patient with ventricular tachycardia. Notice that there is dissociation between His bundle depolarization (H) and ventricular depolarization. In this case the catheters labeled "Abl" and "T" are both within the right ventricle.

arising from the AV node region associated with both retrograde block and bundle branch block aberrancy, and the second is a reentrant circuit using a nodoventricular accessory pathway. Although both of these have been reported in the literature, in practice they are incredibly rare. The best way to rule these unusual arrhythmias out is to identify the presence of dissociation between ventricular signals and His bundle signals. Figure 6.8 shows a young man with wide complex tachycardia. In this case the definitive diagnosis of ventricular tachycardia can be made because of the presence of dissociation between ventricular electrograms and the His electrograms. This finding confirms that any structures at the His bundle or "above" (AV node, atria) are not required for maintenance of tachycardia.

The situation is much more difficult in the setting of a 1 : 1 ventricular and atrial relationship. There are several strategies that can be tried, but the most commonly used approach is to use adenosine to produce retrograde block within the AV node and evaluate whether the wide complex tachycardia terminates. Continuation of wide complex tachycardia in the presence of transient ventriculoatrial block establishes the likely diagnosis of ventricular tachycardia (Fig. 6.9).

Initiation and termination

As will be discussed in Chapter 14, the method for induction and termination of ventricular tachycardia provides clues for the mechanism of tachycardia. Most patients with structural heart disease due to myocardial infarction develop ventricular tachycardia caused by reentrant circuits that use protected channels of viable tissue within scar. Premature beats will block in one portion of the channel, propagate slowly in another channel, and set up a reentrant circuit. The ability to induce a ventricular arrhythmia with premature ventricular

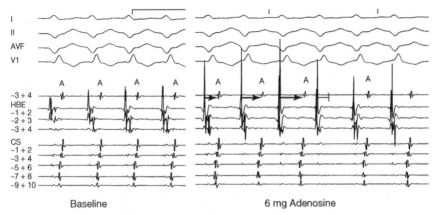

Baseline   6 mg Adenosine

Figure 6.9 Patient with wide complex tachycardia with a right bundle branch block morphology (positive QRS in V_1) and 1 : 1 ventriculoatrial conduction. Earliest atrial activation is observed in the His bundle electrograms (HBE). After infusion with adenosine, retrograde ventriculoatrial Wenckebach block is produced (progressively lengthening arrows culminating in block). Continuation of the tachycardia despite the presence of ventriculoatrial block confirms the presence of ventricular tachycardia.

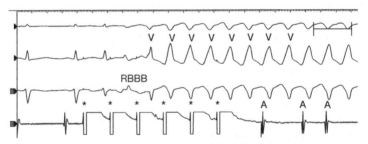

Figure 6.10 Rapid atrial pacing (*) first yields a positive QRS in V_1 (right bundle branch block morphology, RBBB), but quickly a wide complex tachycardia with a left bundle branch block morphology (negative QRS in V_1) is induced. When atrial pacing is stopped, the presence of atrioventricular dissociation confirms the presence of ventricular tachycardia.

beats strongly suggests reentry as a mechanism. In contrast, automatic ventricular tachycardias often require infusion with a beta-agonist (isoproterenol is usually used in the electrophysiology laboratory) and are related to high ventricular rate either by atrial pacing or by ventricular pacing. Figure 6.10 shows a patient who has wide complex tachycardia initiated with atrial pacing. Atrial pacing first induces a beat with right bundle branch block (positive QRS complex in V_1). However, a wide complex tachycardia with a wide negative QRS complex in V_1 (left bundle branch block morphology) is then induced. When atrial pacing is stopped, the presence of atrioventricular dissociation confirms the presence of ventricular tachycardia.

In the presence of a 1 : 1 ventriculoatrial relationship it can be difficult to determine the specific form of supraventricular tachycardia once ventricular tachycardia has been "ruled out." In general, the clinician performs various pacing maneuvers similar to those discussed in the previous chapter, such as placing timed premature ventricular or atrial contractions when the His bundle is refractory.

CHAPTER 7

New technology

The last few years have seen a remarkable technological revolution in the electrophysiology laboratory, with the development and application of new tools for intracardiac imaging and mapping. Although the details and clinical uses of these technologies are beyond the scope of this introductory text, it is important to have at least a rudimentary understanding of the newer technologies that increasingly play an important role in all electrophysiology laboratories.

Intracardiac echocardiography

Miniaturization of ultrasound technology has allowed ultrasound transducers to be mounted on disposable catheters to allow for real-time imaging from within the heart. There are two types of intracardiac echocardiographic catheters available. Phased array transducers use an electronic system that really is like a miniaturized transesophageal echocardiography probe. Phased array transducers allow color flow and monitoring of Doppler. In addition, because of the frequencies used for imaging, cardiac and extracardiac structures 4–5 cm from the probe can be visualized very clearly. The catheters are deflectable in multiple planes, allowing the complete visual exploration of almost any region of interest.

Mechanical transducers use a small piezoelectric crystal that rotates rapidly on a shaft. Mechanical transducers have superb near-field imaging characteristics but are limited by lack of Doppler and poor visualization of "distant" structures. One important use for mechanical transducers is that combined echocardiography and fluoroscopy can help identify the location of anatomic structures quite accurately. For example, in Chapter 1, the interatrial septum is located by intracardiac echocardiography and one simply moves the tip of the Mullins sheath to that exact position.

Regardless of technique, intracardiac echocardography can be very useful during electrophysiologic studies for identifying potential complications. Figure 7.1 shows a small physiologic pericardial effusion at the superior vena cava–right atrial junction. Continuous real-time evaluation during an electrophysiologic study allows for identification of an enlarging pericardial effusion. Another use for intracardiac echocardiography is identification of intraatrial thrombi. In Fig. 7.2, a mobile echogenic structure that most likely represents an

Understanding Intracardiac EGMs and ECGs. By Fred Kusumoto. Published 2010 by Blackwell Publishing. ISBN: 978-1-4051-8410-6

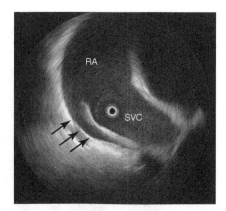

Figure 7.1 Intracardiac echocardiography showing a small pericardial effusion (arrows). RA, right atrium; SVC, superior vena cava.

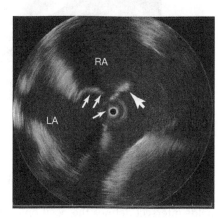

Figure 7.2 Intracardiac echocardiography showing the presence of a thrombus (large arrow) attached to the interatrial septum (small arrows). RA, right atrium; LA, left atrium.

intracardiac thrombus attached to the interatrial septum was identified during electrophysiology testing.

Catheter location/mapping systems

Just over a decade ago, the introduction of systems that allow the operator to locate a catheter in three-dimensional space revolutionized the field of electrophysiology and ablation. Instead or relying on two-dimensional fluoroscopic images to locate catheters within the heart, clinicians could evaluate electrograms associated with a specific position, identify and tag important anatomic points or identify regions of interest, and return to those points at any time within the study.

Magnetic positioning

The first commercially available catheter location and mapping system uses a locator pad placed underneath the upper back of the patient. The pad has three coils that generate a constant magnetic field that decays as the distance

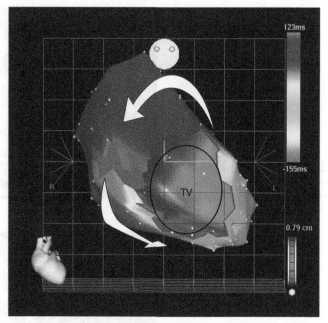

Figure 7.3 Endocardial activation map of atrial flutter using a magnetic positioning catheter. TV, tricuspid valve. (Image courtesy of Biosense Webster (Jeff Bennett).)

from each coil increases. A sensor embedded in the catheter tip measures the strength of each magnetic field, and the point where these three magnetic fields intersect defines the position of the catheter. The system has been validated to approximately 1 cm by clinical studies.

Combining known positioning information with electrogram timing to a fiduciary point allows an activation map to be produced of the chamber of interest. Similarly, the course of a reentrant circuit can be easily identified. Although it can be difficult to appreciate with black and white images, Fig. 7.3 shows an endocardial activation map of reentrant atrial flutter circling around the tricuspid valve. In the newest iterations of these systems, electrophysiologic information can be combined with images obtained from cardiac CT or intracardiac echocardiography (Fig. 7.4). Integration of information from different sources holds promise for revolutionizing the field of electrophysiology.

Noncontact mapping

When a three-dimensional space is placed within another three-dimensional space, if the electrical potential on one surface is measured the electrical potential on the second surface can be determined. This technology is combined with a locator system that can locate any catheter using a low-current locator signal through the tip of any electrode of interest to the reference electrode.

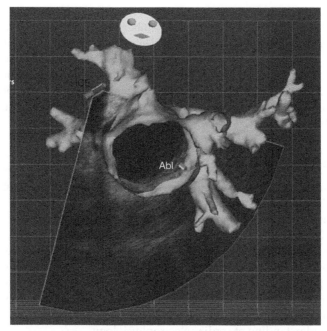

Figure 7.4 Integration of intracardiac echocardiography (ICE) imaging with computed tomography imaging and real-time positioning of a mapping catheter (Abl).
(Image courtesy of Biosense Webster (Jeff Bennett).)

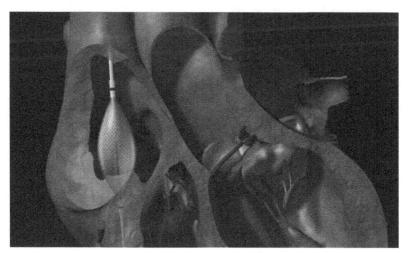

Figure 7.5 Balloon catheter placed in the right atrium. (Image courtesy of Glen Greenberg, St. Jude Medical.)

When using a noncontact system, a saline-filled balloon covered by a mesh of electrodes is inflated in the chamber of interest (Fig. 7.5). This can generate up to 3000 virtual endocardial electrograms, which can be integrated by computer algorithms to generate a simple visual picture of cardiac depolarization. A mapping electrode can then be moved over the endocardial surface to produce a shell that can be used to display the cardiac depolarization information. Specific structures within the shell can be tagged (pulmonary veins, valve orifices).

Robotic navigation

Several commercially available devices are available that can assist catheter ablation. The first uses two focused field magnets that generate a magnetic field around a patient's torso. The clinician can then steer specially designed very flexible magnetic catheters to different portions of the heart by manipulating the magnetic field. A second system uses a conventional catheter that is placed within two steerable sheaths. The operator uses a joystick control to carefully position the catheter to the desired location. Both of these systems hold promise for aiding catheter positioning, but their clinical utility remains unproven, and the introduction of such systems will not supplant the necessity of a firm understanding of cardiac electrophysiology.

CHAPTER 8

Power sources for ablation

For the first 20 years, electrophysiologic studies served diagnostic purposes only. This changed in the 1980s with the development of techniques to ablate the His bundle or specific arrhythmia substrates using high-energy shocks, using a defibrillator to deliver an electric shock directly to the catheter tip. Although effective, direct-current energy required general anesthesia, was all-or-none, and did not produce reliable and "controllable" lesions. As an alternative, radiofrequency energy had been used for many years in the operating room as an energy source to cauterize tissue, and this was applied to electrophysiology procedures in the late 1980s and early 1990s. More recently cryothermal energy, used by surgeons for many years in the operating room, has been introduced as an important power source in the electrophysiology laboratory.

Radiofrequency energy

Radiofrequency energy has been used for over a century to produce surgical lesions. Current generators in use in electrophysiology laboratories produce alternating-current energy with a cycle length of 300–750 kHz. For comparison, frequencies between 88 and 110 kHz are used for transmission of FM radio signals.

Radiofrequency energy makes lesions through heating from the relatively small surface electrode. Electromagnetic energy is converted into mechanical movement of cellular molecules with production of heat. This type of heating is called resistive or ohmic heating. Multiple experimental studies have shown that irreversible cell death occurs at temperatures greater than 50 °C. Very little tissue injury occurs below 45 °C. Temperature decreases rapidly from the catheter-tip electrode as the current is dispersed through bodily tissue, so that relatively small lesions, approximately 5–6 mm in diameter and 2–3 mm deep, are produced with standard ablation electrode (4 mm) catheters. Figure 8.1 shows a schematic of energy flow during radiofrequency catheter ablation. A catheter is connected to a radiofrequency generator. The circuit is completed by a large patch placed on the skin. When the catheter tip is placed in contact with the endocardial surface and radiofrequency energy is applied, heating of the tissue occurs, due to the relatively high current density. It is important

Understanding Intracardiac EGMs and ECGs. By Fred Kusumoto. Published 2010 by Blackwell Publishing. ISBN: 978-1-4051-8410-6

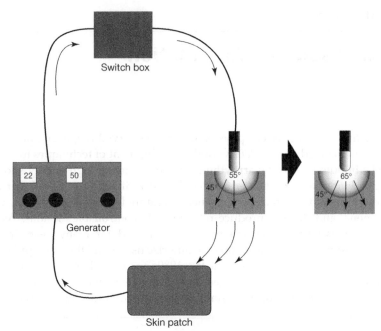

Figure 8.1 Schematic of energy flow during radiofrequency ablation. Application of radiofrequency energy at the catheter tip leads to tissue heating and cellular destruction. Tissue temperatures fall quite rapidly as one moves from the tip outward, thus limiting the size of the lesion. The circuit is completed by a large electrode placed on the skin that returns energy to the generator. When the temperature at the electrode–tissue interface is increased the lesion produced is larger, because more tissue is exposed to temperatures > 50 °C.

to note that if the skin electrode does not have firm contact, skin burns can result, caused by the higher generated current densities at the electrode–skin interface.

Lesion size can be controlled through a number of factors. The most important is temperature at the tissue–electrode interface. Higher temperatures will lead to deeper lesions (Fig. 8.1), because of the larger area with temperatures > 45–50 °C. However, there is a limit to the temperature that can be produced at the catheter tip, since temperatures > 100 °C can lead to boiling and coagulum formation at the tip due to adherence of denatured protein. From the foregoing discussion it is obvious that temperature monitoring during ablation is critical. All modern ablation catheter designs incorporate some method for measuring the temperature of the electrode tip (Fig. 8.2). Radiofrequency generators can deliver varying amounts of power (0–100 watts) to achieve adequate temperature at the ablation site. The amount of power required for a lesion will depend on a number of clinical factors including desired lesion size, ablation tip size, catheter contact, and amount of cooling from blood.

The lesion produced by radiofrequency current is a central zone of coagulation necrosis surrounded by a region of hemorrhage and inflammation. In

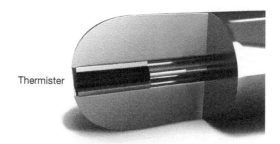

Thermister

Figure 8.2 All modern ablation catheters are designed to monitor temperature from some region of the catheter tip, to provide an estimate of the electrode–tissue interface temperature. (Courtesy of Mike Repshar, Boston Scientific.)

cases where a temperature > 100 °C has been delivered, charred endocardial surface with adherent thrombus can be seen. After several months, fibrous scar, granulation tissue, and other forms of chronic inflammatory response can be observed.

Effectiveness of lesions can be predicted by monitoring impedance. Initially, in the case of an effective lesion production, the impedance will decrease by 5–10 ohms because of tissue swelling. Larger decreases in impedance can be associated with a subsequent impedance rise caused by coagulation formation on the catheter tip. Larger electrodes have the potential for producing larger lesions, because a larger tissue area reaches a temperature greater than 50 °C. Although the standard ablation electrode size is 4 mm, catheters are available with a variety of electrode sizes up to 10 mm. Larger electrodes require more power to generate adequate temperatures. Details of the biophysics of ablation are beyond the scope of this text, but it should be noted that all modern generators are designed to monitor temperature and impedance and to deliver varying amounts of power, and are equipped with a number of automatic options (Fig. 8.3).

Irrigated radiofrequency energy

One method for making larger lesions more quickly is to irrigate the ablation tip with fluid (Fig. 8.4). Cooling the tip "forces" the hotter area deeper, thus potentially making a larger lesion. Cooling of the catheter tip can be achieved using an open system, where saline is flushed through open ports at the electrode tip, or with a closed circulating system. As shown in Fig. 8.5, catheters with larger electrode tend to produce lesions with larger surface areas and catheters with irrigated tips tend to produce deeper lesions. It is important for the clinician to use ablation technique, temperature, electrode size, duration of the lesion, and irrigation to provide the desired lesion size. For example, lesions in ventricular tissue usually require higher temperatures or catheters with larger tips or irrigated tips, while ablations near critical structures such as the AV node are often best performed with smaller electrodes and lower powers.

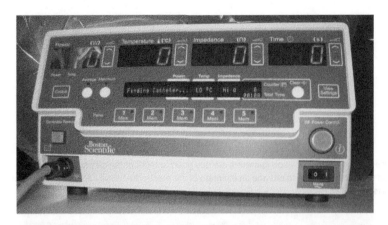

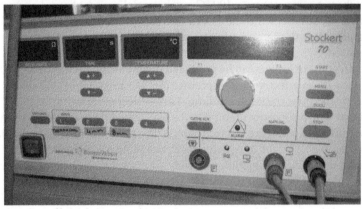

Figure 8.3 Photographs of two commercially available radiofrequency energy generators. Both allow the user to adjust the power delivered and the duration of the ablation with continuous monitoring of impedance and catheter tip temperature.

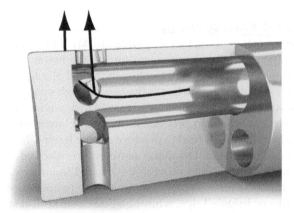

Figure 8.4 Design for an open irrigated ablation catheter. Active pumping of saline cools the tip electrode. (Courtesy of Mike Repshar, Boston Scientific.)

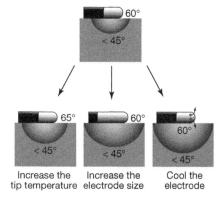

Figure 8.5 In addition to increasing the temperature, lesion size can be increased by increasing the electrode size (as long as the larger electrode is in contact with tissue) or by cooling the tip, which then allows production of higher temperatures deeper below the tissue surface.

Cryothermal energy

Initial arrhythmia surgery in the 1970s used cryothermal energy sources. As tissue is cooled, extracellular and intracellular ice begins to form, which causes disruption of cellular membranes and organelles. In addition to the direct cellular injury, cryothermal energy leads to damage to the microvasculature.

Lesions made with cryothermal energy have several important differences from lesions made with radiofrequency energy. Cryothermal energy will generally produce smaller lesions than radiofrequency energy for a given electrode size. Importantly, cryothermal energy appears to have less endothelial disruption and less activation of molecules that enhance thrombus formation. Cryothermal lesions appear to preserve the extracellular matrix and do not change the tensile strength of ablated tissue. Radiofrequency energy tends to cause denaturation of extracellular proteins and collagen shrinkage, effects that are not observed with cryothermal energy. For these reasons, cryothermal engery has been found to be an excellent power source for lesions that are within or near vascular structures (coronary sinus, pulmonary veins). Cryothermal energy may also be useful for ablation within the pericardial space.

Specific Arrhythmias

PART 2

Specific Arrhythmias

CHAPTER 9

Accessory pathways

The existence of multiple connections between the atrium and ventricle was first proposed by Kent in the late nineteenth century, although by the early twentieth century the AV node and His bundle had been identified as the pathway that electrically connected the atria to the ventricles. The concept that additional muscular connections between atria and ventricle existed was controversial until 1942, when Wood and colleagues described the first histologic evidence of three accessory pathways connecting the right atrium and right ventricle in a young boy who died suddenly. The properties of accessory pathways have fascinated electrophysiologists for many years, particularly after seminal work by Sealy, Scheinman, and others that reported successful surgical and catheter-based ablation techniques to eliminate accessory pathways.

Anatomy and electrophysiology

The AV node generally forms the only connection between atrial and ventricular tissue, with the remainder of the atrial tissue and ventricular tissue separated by the fibrous annulus that forms the scaffolding for the mitral and aortic valves. This arrangement, along with the refractory properties of the AV node and His bundle, reduces the likelihood of "feedback" between atrial and ventricular depolarization. There is a small but definite incidence of sudden cardiac death in patients with accessory pathways, particularly in those patients with symptomatic arrhythmias (2%). It is more controversial whether asymptomatic patients share this magnitude of risk for sudden cardiac death.

The electrophysiologic properties of accessory pathways can vary significantly (Table 9.1). Most commonly accessory pathways are composed of tissue histologically and electrophysiologically like atrial or ventricular tissue, with a rapid phase 0 upstroke and a plateau phase. Accessory pathways can usually conduct in both directions, from atrium to ventricle and from ventricle to atrium. However, some accessory pathways can only conduct in one direction, usually from ventricle to atrium. These accessory pathways are often called "concealed," because their presence is not observed during sinus rhythm (no atrioventricular activation) but they can participate in supraventricular tachycardia because of robust ventricle-to-atrium depolarization. Some accessory pathways conduct very slowly, more like AV node tissue.

Understanding Intracardiac EGMs and ECGs. By Fred Kusumoto. Published 2010 by Blackwell Publishing. ISBN: 978-1-4051-8410-6

Table 9.1 Atrioventricular accessory pathway types.

Location	ECG characteristics
Normal conduction properties	
Manifest	Accessory pathway conducts in both directions
	Delta wave and a short PR interval will be observed during sinus rhythm
	Supraventricular tachycardia is most common, although regular and irregular wide complex tachycardia may be observed
Concealed	Accessory pathway only conducts "backwards" from ventricle to atria
	The QRS during sinus rhythm will be normal
	Supraventricular tachycardia will be the predominant tachycardia
Anterograde only	Accessory pathway conducts only from the atria to the ventricles
	Short PR with a delta wave will be observed during sinus rhythm
Slow conduction properties	
Anterograde only	Normal ECG at baseline (slow conduction does not produce a delta wave)
	Present with wide complex tachycardia
Retrograde only	Permanent junctional reciprocating tachycardia (PJRT)
	Incessant supraventricular tachycardia

ECG findings in patients with accessory pathways

ECG during sinus rhythm (delta waves)

The ECG is the single most important noninvasive tool for identifying the presence of an accessory pathway. Patients with accessory pathways that can conduct in the anterograde direction will have abnormal QRS complexes that are often referred to as "manifest" or "preexcited." These terms simply mean that the presence of an accessory pathway can be identified because a portion of the ventricles is depolarized early or "preexcited" due to accessory pathway depolarization. In these patients, the ventricle is activated by both the AV node and the accessory pathway, and the QRS morphology can provide important clues for the location of the accessory pathway.

Remember from Chapter 2 that ordinarily the AV node is characterized by slow conduction, and the right and left ventricles depolarize almost simultaneously. In a patient with a right-sided accessory pathway connecting the right atrium and the right ventricle, the wave of depolarization over the accessory pathway "bypasses" the AV node and a portion of the right ventricle is depolarized early (Fig. 9.1). This leads to an absent isoelectric PR interval and an abnormal QRS complex that is wide and has a slurred upstoke or "delta" wave. The delta wave is caused by early activation of the right ventricle,

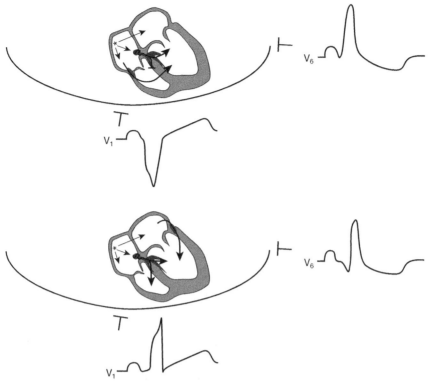

Figure 9.1 Schematic showing the effects of a right-sided and a left-sided accessory pathway on the baseline surface ECG. *Top:* In the presence of a right-sided accessory pathway, a large portion of the right ventricle is activated very early (due to proximity of the accessory pathway to the sinus node), leading to the absence of an isoelectric PR interval and a predominantly negative and wide QRS complex in V_1. *Bottom:* In the presence of a left-sided accessory pathway early activation of the left ventricle leads to a prominent R wave in V_1. A short isoelectric PR segment is often observed before the delta wave because depolarization of the AV node occurs before depolarization of the accessory pathway. However, because of the rapid conduction properties of the accessory pathway a delta wave is still present.

and the QRS complex is wide because the right ventricle depolarized by the accessory pathway proceeds by slower cell-to-cell depolarization that does not use the specialized His–Purkinje tissue. Since the right ventricle is activated before the left ventricle, the general shape of the QRS complex looks similar to the QRS in left bundle branch block (in which there is delayed left ventricular depolarization). The QRS complex will be negative in V_1 and positive in the lateral leads V_5, V_6, I, and aVL. From Fig. 9.1 it can be seen that the initial part of the QRS complex is due to depolarization via the accessory pathway and the middle and later parts of the QRS are due to depolarization of both the accessory pathway and the AV node. A 12-lead ECG from a patient with a right-sided accessory pathway is shown in Fig. 9.2. Notice that the P wave and QRS

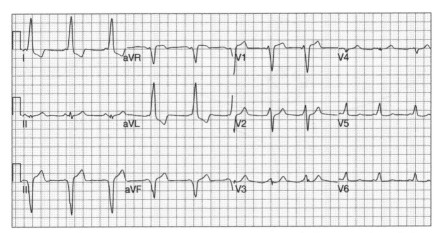

Figure 9.2 ECG from a patient with a right-sided accessory pathway. (Reprinted with permission from Kusumoto FM. *ECG Interpretation: From Pathophysiology to Clinical Application*. New York, NY: Springer, 2009.)

complex are not separated by an isoelectric PR segment. The QRS complex in lead V_1 is predominantly negative, because of early right-to-left depolarization of the right ventricle due to the right-sided accessory pathway.

Patients with a left-sided accessory pathway will have a different ECG pattern. In this case a short isoelectric PR interval may be observed, since the AV node will be depolarized before the accessory pathway (think of it "getting a head start"). However, since the AV node has slow conduction properties, depolarization via the accessory pathway still "beats" the AV node and a delta wave and an abnormal QRS complex are still seen. In this case left ventricular activation occurs before right ventricular activation, and the general shape of the QRS complex will resemble a right bundle branch block pattern with a prominent positive QRS in V_1. Since the delta wave represents ventricular depolarization via the accessory pathway, careful analysis of the delta wave can provide further clues for accessory pathway localization. If the accessory pathway is located at the lateral wall of the mitral annulus, the delta wave will be negative in I and aVL due to ventricular depolarization traveling away from this area (Fig. 9.3). If the accessory pathway is located more inferiorly and closer to the septum (Fig. 9.4) the delta waves will be negative in the inferior leads (II, III, and aVF).

In patients with a "concealed" accessory pathway a normal PR interval will be present and a delta wave will not be observed since there is no anterograde conduction over the accessory pathway. It has been suggested that some pathways are concealed because they are thinner and the voltage generated by accessory pathway depolarization is not sufficient to depolarize adjacent ventricular tissue. However, since the atria are thinner, retrograde depolarization of atrial tissue can still occur, and for this reason these patients still develop supraventricular tachycardia.

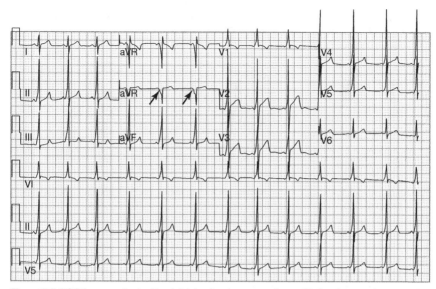

Figure 9.3 ECG from a patient with a left lateral accessory pathway. Notice the prominent positive QRS complex in V$_1$. Since the accessory pathway inserts into the lateral left ventricle, the delta wave is negative in aVL (arrows).

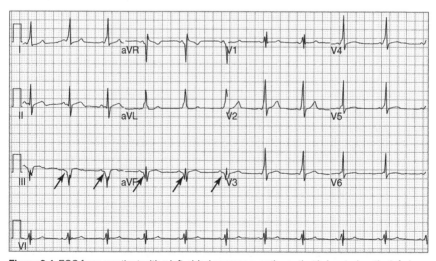

Figure 9.4 ECG from a patient with a left-sided accessory pathway that is located on the inferior portion of the mitral annulus. Since the pathway is left-sided a prominent positive QRS complex is seen in lead V$_1$. However, the delta waves are negative in III and aVF (arrows). (Reprinted with permission from Kusumoto FM. *ECG Interpretation: From Pathophysiology to Clinical Application*. New York, NY: Springer, 2009.)

Orthodromic AV reentrant tachycardia	Antidromic AV reentrant tachycardia	Atrial tachycardia with rapid anterograde conduction
	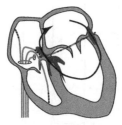	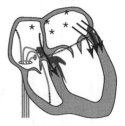
Regular narrow complex tachycardia	Regular wide complex tachycardia	Irregular very rapid wide complex tachycardia

Figure 9.5 Types of tachycardia that can develop in patients with an accessory pathway. The most commonly observed arrhythmia is orthodromic AV reentrant tachycardia (orthodromic AVRT), in which a reentrant circuit develops that travels in the normal atrioventricular direction over the AV node and retrogradely over the accessory pathway. The rarest arrhythmia is antidromic AV reentrant tachycardia, in which the reentrant circuit is reversed with anterograde activation over the accessory pathway and retrograde over the AV node. This leads to a regular wide complex tachycardia, since the ventricles are not activated via the His–Purkinje tissue. The third type of arrhythmia that can develop is atrial fibrillation or some other types of atrial arrhythmia that lead to rapid ventricular activation via the accessory pathway.

ECG during tachycardias involving accessory pathways

Patients with accessory pathways can often have associated tachycardias. This association was first described in the early years of the twentieth century, but the most complete discussion of ventricular preexcitation and associated tachycardias was published by Wolff, Parkinson, and White in 1930, and for this reason the presence of a delta wave on ECG and accompanying episodes of rapid heart rate is usually called the Wolff–Parkinson–White syndrome.

Three types of arrhythmias can develop in the presence of an accessory pathway (Fig. 9.5). The most common type of tachycardia is *orthodromic atrioventricular reentrant tachycardia* (orthodromic AVRT), in which a reentrant circuit develops that activates the AV node in the normal fashion (*ortho* is Greek for regular), and, after activating ventricular tissue, the wave of depolarization travels retrogradely over the accessory pathway to depolarize the atria. Since there is sequential activation of the ventricles and atria, think of two alternately blinking lights: this arrhythmia is often described as reciprocating or "circus movement" (this historical term has been used to describe any tachycardia due to reentry – similar to a "pony running around a circus ring"). The ECG during orthodromic reciprocating tachycardia will display a regular narrow complex tachycardia, because the ventricles are activated normally via the AV node. In some cases the presence of a retrograde P wave can be seen in the ST segment (Fig. 9.6). Even for experienced ECG readers, determining the location and shape of the P wave during tachycardia can be very difficult. As discussed in the

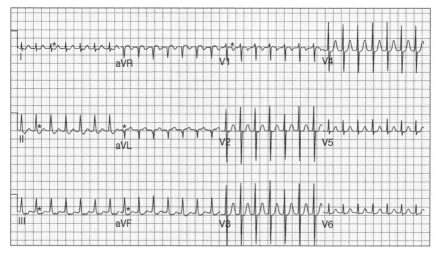

Figure 9.6 ECG during orthodromic AVRT. Notice the P waves in the ST segments (*). (Reprinted with permission from Kusumoto FM. *ECG Interpretation: From Pathophysiology to Clinical Application*. New York, NY: Springer, 2009.)

subsequent section, one of the main advantages of electrophysiologic testing is unequivocal information on the timing and pattern of atrial depolarization.

Patients can also develop *antidromic atrioventricular reentrant tachycardia* (antidromic reciprocating tachycardia), in which the direction of the reentrant circuit is reversed and the ventricles are activated via the accessory pathway and the atria are activated by the AV node. Antidromic reciprocating tachycardia is characterized by a regular wide complex tachycardia (since the ventricles are depolarized by the accessory pathway). Sustained antidromic tachycardia is very rare.

Finally, patients can develop *atrial fibrillation* with rapid ventricular activation. Normally, in the presence of a rapid atrial tachycardia of any kind, the slow conduction properties of the AV node act to "protect" the ventricles from rapid rates. However, if atrial fibrillation develops in the presence of an accessory pathway, the ventricles can be depolarized very rapidly. In fact the triad of an irregular, very fast, wide complex rhythm should always arouse suspicion for the presence of an accessory pathway and atrial fibrillation. Figure 9.7 shows the ECG from the same patient shown in Fig. 9.4 during evaluation in the emergency department, where he was complaining of light-headedness and a rapid heart rate. The accessory pathway can permit very rapid ventricular depolarization. It is generally agreed by most investigators that sudden death occurs in patients with accessory pathways because of rapid ventricular activation from atrial fibrillation initiating ventricular fibrillation. This is the reason that increased risk for sudden death is not observed in those patients that have concealed accessory pathways (no delta waves noted during sinus rhythm).

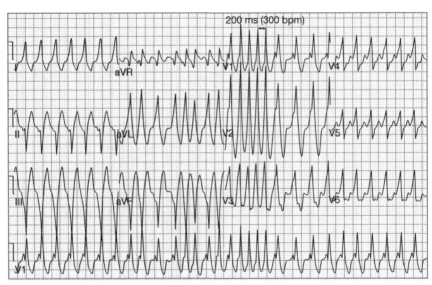

Figure 9.7 ECG from the same patient as Fig. 9.4. Notice that some QRS complexes are separated by only 200 ms (a heart rate of 300 beats per minute). The triad of an irregular wide complex tachycardia with the presence of very short RR intervals should always arouse suspicion for atrial fibrillation with rapid depolarization due to the presence of an accessory pathway. (Reprinted with permission from Kusumoto FM. *ECG Interpretation: From Pathophysiology to Clinical Application.* New York, NY: Springer, 2009.)

Electrophysiologic testing

Baseline evaluation

Electrophysiology studies can help delineate the properties of accessory pathways and evaluate risk for sudden cardiac death and mechanisms of arrhythmia initiation. At baseline, the HV interval will be very short and in some cases negative. The baseline electrograms in a patient with an accessory pathway are shown in Fig. 9.8. The patient is in sinus rhythm, with the earliest atrial signal observed in the high right atrium (HRA). Notice that the PR interval is significantly shortened and that the beginning of the QRS (dotted line) actually precedes His bundle depolarization (H) for a negative HV interval. Earliest ventricular activation (V) is observed in the coronary sinus catheter (electrode 3,4). This suggests that the patient has a left sided-accessory pathway. Notice that the QRS complex is also consistent with a left-sided accessory pathway, with a prominent positive QRS complex recorded in lead V_1. The intracardiac electrogram recordings reinforce the concept that in the presence of an accessory pathway the ventricles are depolarized by both the accessory pathway and the AV node/His bundle system, and that the initial portion of the QRS complex represents ventricular depolarization over the accessory pathway.

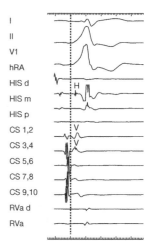

Figure 9.8 Baseline electrograms in a patient with an accessory pathway. Notice that the beginning of the QRS (dotted line) actually precedes depolarization of the His bundle (H).

Effect of atrial pacing on ventricular depolarization

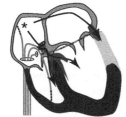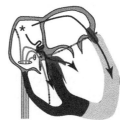

Figure 9.9 Schematic showing the effect of atrial pacing on the QRS morphology in a patient with an accessory pathway. As the pacing rate is increased (left panel), decremental conduction in the AV node leads to more ventricular depolarization via the accessory pathway relative to the AV node. For this reason the QRS complex often becomes more wider and bizarre appearing.

Atrial pacing

With progressively more rapid atrial pacing, the delta wave will become more prominent as more of the ventricle is activated via the accessory pathway (Fig. 9.9). Remember that the normal response of the AV node to atrial pacing is slowed conduction. Slower conduction over the AV node means that more of the ventricle is depolarized via the accessory pathway. With more rapid atrial pacing the observed response will depend on the relative refractory properties of the AV node and the accessory pathway. If the refractory period in the accessory pathway is reached first, the QRS will suddenly normalize due to conduction down the AV node alone. As the atrial pacing rate is increased, and the refractory period of the AV node is reached, eventually an atrial paced beat without a QRS complex will be seen. In contrast, if the AV node blocks first, sometimes one will observe a variable QRS complex due to different proportions of the ventricle being depolarized via the accessory pathway, but

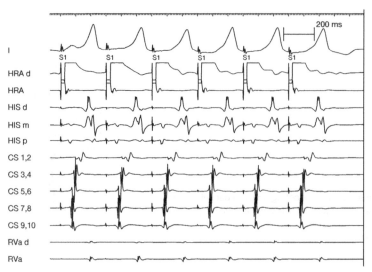

Figure 9.10 Atrial pacing in a patient with an accessory pathway. Atrial stimuli (S$_1$) are delivered at 300 ms intervals (200 beats per minute). The accessory pathway conducts in 1 : 1 fashion.

eventually, as the atrial pacing rate is increased, dropped QRS complexes will be observed due to block in the accessory pathway (without an intervening period of normal QRS complexes). Again, the response observed for a specific patient will depend on the relative conduction properties of the accessory pathway and the AV node. Examples of both responses are shown for two patients in Figs. 9.10 through 9.13.

The response of an accessory pathway to atrial pacing for the first patient is shown in Figs. 9.10 through 9.12. In Fig. 9.10, atrial pacing from the high right atrium is performed at a cycle length of 300 ms. Every pacing stimulus is followed by an atrial signal and a ventricular signal. In Fig. 9.11, when the pacing stimuli are delivered at shorter intervals (250 ms), although every pacing stimulus is associated with an atrial signal (A), a QRS complex and ventricular signal is observed for every second atrial stimulus (2 : 1 block in the accessory pathway). In this case the AV node blocked earlier so the atrial signal is not followed by a QRS complex. This is the usual circumstance where the refractory period of the accessory pathway is significantly shorter than the refractory period of the AV node. This is the electrophysiologic "proof" that accessory pathways allow more rapid ventricular activation than the AV node. The development of 2 : 1 block allows the astute clinician to differentiate between signals due to atrial activity and ventricular activity. In the CS 3,4 recording one can see that the low-frequency "hump" (arrow in Fig. 9.11) is only observed with ventricular depolarization, while the high-frequency "spikes" due to atrial depolarization are seen after every stimulus. Notice that the earliest ventricular signal is observed in CS 3,4, suggesting that the accessory pathway is located near these electrodes. The closer one paces to the atrial insertion

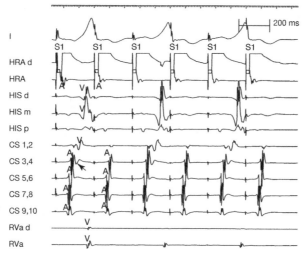

Figure 9.11 Atrial pacing in the same patient as Fig. 9.10 with stimuli (S_1) now delivered at 250 ms intervals. The accessory pathway conducts with 2 : 1 block (every second atrial signal (A) leads to ventricular depolarization (V). Since the AV node refractory period has already been reached, the blocked atrial beat does not result in a QRS complex. The development of 2 : 1 block allows the clinician to determine that low-frequency signals (humps rather than spikes) in the coronary sinus recordings are due to ventricular depolarization (arrow).

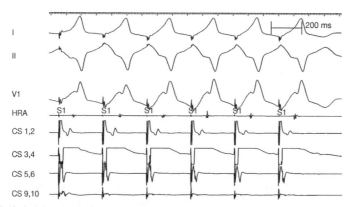

Figure 9.12 Atrial pacing in the same patient as Figs. 9.10 and 9.11. This time pacing stimuli are delivered at 300 ms intervals from the coronary sinus electrodes 3,4. Since pacing is now performed near the site of the accessory pathway, the stimulus to the onset of the QRS is very short; the upstroke of the QRS starts just after the pacing stimulus.

point of the accessory pathway, the shorter the interval between the stimulus and the onset of the QRS. This phenomenon is illustrated in Fig. 9.12. Pacing is performed from the coronary sinus electrodes 3,4 at a pacing interval of 300 ms. Although the QRS complex is similar to the QRS complex in Fig. 9.10, the interval between the stimulus and the onset of the QRS is very short, since

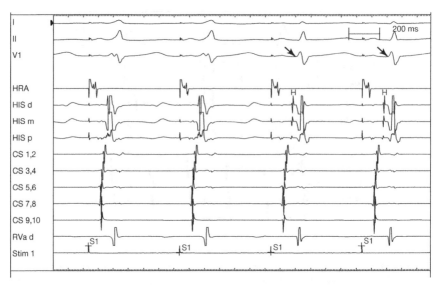

Figure 9.13 Atrial pacing at an interval of 600 ms (100 beats per minute). During pacing there is sudden normalization of the QRS complex (arrow) associated with a His bundle electrogram (H) due to block in the accessory pathway.

atrial pacing is performed near the site of the accessory pathway eliminating any delay due to depolarization of atrial tissue between the stimulation site and the accessory pathway.

Figure 9.13 shows the effects of atrial pacing for the second patient with an accessory pathway. In this case, atrial pacing at an interval of 600 ms leads to intermittent block in the accessory pathway, resulting in normalization of the QRS complex and a distinct His electrogram recorded in the His catheter. In this case the His bundle recording was obscured by ventricular depolarization. In this patient the anterograde refractory period of the accessory pathway is longer than the anterograde refractory period of the AV node, and when the accessory pathway blocks conduction to the ventricles can still occur over the AV node. This finding suggests that the accessory pathway cannot conduct very well in the anterograde direction (since it is already blocking).

In addition to pacing the atria at a constant rate, full electrophysiologic evaluation of the accessory pathway requires evaluation of the response to atrial premature beats. Usually, with earlier and earlier atrial extrastimuli, pre-excitation will increase and the QRS will become wider. Since earlier premature atrial beats will lead to slower conduction in the AV node and a longer AH interval, the His signal will often become obscured by the ventricular signal as the atrial extrastimulus is coupled earlier and earlier. When, the refractory period of the accessory pathway is reached, the QRS will suddenly normalize. However, if the refractory period of the accessory pathway is shorter than the refractory period of the AV node, when the premature atrial complex blocks in the accessory pathway, no QRS complex will be observed.

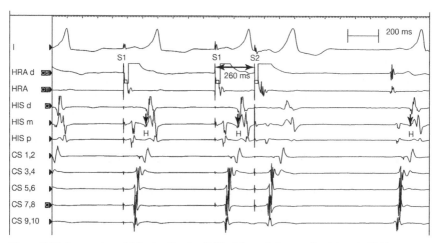

Figure 9.14 A premature atrial extrastimulus (S_2) is delivered at a coupling interval of 260 ms. A His bundle signal (H, arrow) noted during the drive train (S_1) and in sinus rhythm is not observed with the premature beat.

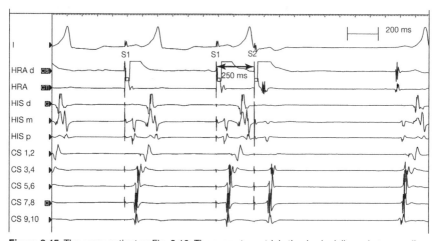

Figure 9.15 The same patient as Fig. 9.13. The premature atrial stimulus is delivered at a coupling interval of 250 ms, resulting in block in the accessory pathway. The refractory period of the accessory pathway is 250 ms.

In Fig. 9.14, a premature atrial stimulus at a coupling interval of 260 ms is delivered. Conduction via the accessory pathway is present, and a wide QRS complex is associated with the premature atrial stimulus. Notice though that no His bundle signal (H) accompanies the premature atrial stimulus. Although this could be due to delay in the AV node and the His signal being obscured by the ventricular signal, more likely block in the AV node has occurred, since with a shorter coupling interval of 250 ms the refractory period of the accessory pathway is reached (Fig. 9.15). Determining the refractory period of the accessory pathway can help determine the risk for sudden cardiac death. Patients with accessory pathways who develop sudden cardiac death often have a shorter accessory pathway refractory period, since a shorter refractory period means that more rapid ventricular depolarization can occur. Most experts suggest that risk of sudden cardiac death is increased in those patients with accessory pathway refractory periods of less than 270 ms. A useful analogy is to think of the accessory pathway and the AV node as two roads that connect two cities (the atria and the ventricles). An accessory pathway with a short refractory period is like a freeway that can allow many cars (or impulses) to travel to the ventricle, leading to "too many cars" (rapid ventricular rates and possible development of ventricular fibrillation). An accessory pathway with a long anterograde refractory period, as shown in Fig. 9.13, is unlikely to lead to rapid ventricular rates, and this patient is probably at very low risk for sudden cardiac death.

Ventricular pacing

With ventricular pacing in a patient with an accessory pathway, retrograde depolarization of the atria can occur via two routes: the AV node and the accessory pathway. The activation pattern of the atrial electrograms can provide clues to how retrograde activation is occurring. Figures 9.16 and 9.17 show the typical response to ventricular pacing in a patient with an accessory pathway.

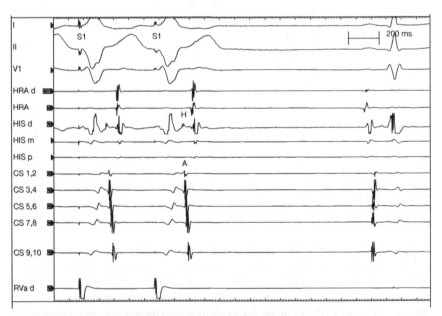

Figure 9.16 Ventricular pacing at a constant rate of 600 ms (S₁) produces a 1 : 1 atrial response. Earliest atrial activation is observed in the lateral wall of the left atrium (CS 1,2) suggesting that the patient has a left lateral accessory pathway. Evidence for continued retrograde activation via the His bundle is suggested by the presence of a discrete His signal (H).

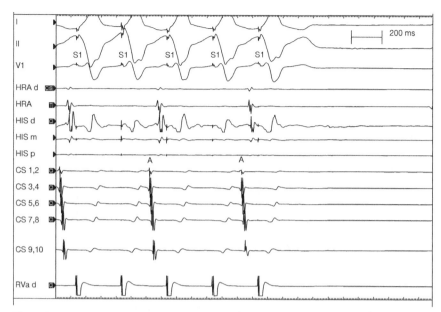

Figure 9.17 The same patient as in Fig. 9.16, but now pacing at a shorter interval (300 ms). In this case 2 : 1 retrograde block in the accessory pathway is observed. There is no evidence for conduction via the His bundle: no His signals are recorded, and there is no evidence of early atrial activation in the catheter located at the interatrial septum, the His catheter.

In Fig. 9.16 ventricular pacing at a constant stimulation interval of 600 ms results in an atrial activation pattern with the earliest atrial signal in the distal coronary sinus (CS 1,2). It would be very unusual for retrograde conduction via the AV node to have earliest atrial activation in the lateral wall of the left atrium. Retrograde atrial activation that appears to emanate from a spot that is located away from the septum (the expected spot for retrograde conduction via the AV node) is called "eccentric" atrial depolarization. While not absolute, the presence of eccentric retrograde atrial activation during ventricular pacing should always arouse suspicion for a second path other than the His bundle/ AV node connecting the ventricles and the atria. In Fig. 9.16 evidence for continued retrograde depolarization of the His bundle is present, since a discrete His electrogram is recorded. Figure 9.17 shows the same patient as Fig. 9.16, but now with pacing at a shorter interval (300 ms). In this case there is 2 : 1 retrograde block in the accessory pathway, as every other S_1 yields an atrial signal. In this case there is no evidence of His depolarization (no His signal is observed).

With premature ventricular stimulation, the retrograde properties of the accessory pathway can be evaluated. In Fig. 9.18, a premature ventricular stimulus delivered at a coupling interval of 260 ms produces an eccentric atrial activation pattern with initial atrial activation in the distal coronary sinus due to the presence of a left lateral accessory pathway. Notice that during the

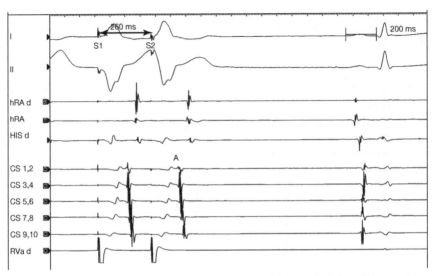

Figure 9.18 After a ventricular pacing train, a single ventricular stimulus is delivered at a coupling interval of 260 ms. Eccentric retrograde atrial activation is observed with the earliest atrial signal noted in the distal coronary sinus (CS 1,2). Notice that for the sinus beat after cessation of pacing the QRS complex is normal without a delta wave. This is a patient with a concealed accessory pathway that does not conduct in the anterograde direction. It is thought that concealed pathways are so thin they do not generate enough current for adjacent ventricular cells to depolarize but can generate enough current to depolarize atrial tissue.

sinus beat after ventricular pacing is stopped, the QRS complex has a normal pattern. This is an example of a patient with a concealed accessory pathway that conducts only in the retrograde direction (reexamine Fig. 9.16). In Fig. 9.19, with an earlier premature ventricular stimulus at 250 ms, a QRS is noted but no atrial electrograms. In this case the retrograde refractory period of the accessory pathway is 250 ms.

Tachycardia

As noted above, the most commonly observed tachycardia encountered in a patient with an accessory pathway is orthodromic AVRT. Figure 9.20 shows initiation of orthodromic AVRT with a premature atrial contraction (S_2). The premature atrial contraction leads to delay within the AV node (prolonged AH interval), and retrograde atrial activation occurs in the distal coronary sinus (CS 3,4) located in the lateral wall of the left atrium, and reentry is initiated. Notice that the patient probably has a concealed accessory pathway, since the QRS complex during the pacing train is the same as the QRS complex during tachycardia.

When tachycardia is initiated in a patient with an accessory pathway it is important for the clinician to perform the pacing maneuvers discussed in Chapter 5. Simply because a patient has an accessory pathway does not

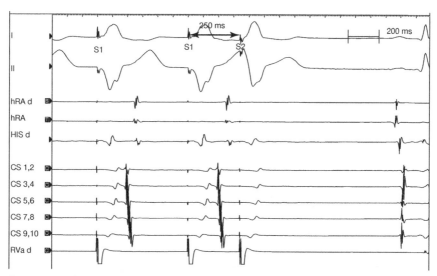

Figure 9.19 In the same patient as Fig. 9.18, when the ventricular coupling interval is decreased to 250 ms a QRS complex without an accompanying atrial signal is recorded, because of retrograde block in the accessory pathway. The retrograde refractory period of the accessory pathway would be calculated to be 250 ms.

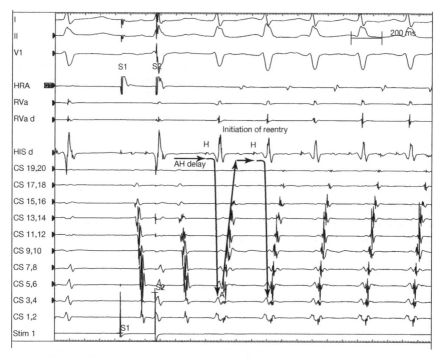

Figure 9.20 Initiation of orthodromic atrioventricular reentrant tachycardia. A premature atrial contraction (S_2) results in slow conduction in the AV node (AH interval prolongation). The wave of depolarization travels through ventricular tissue and then back retrogradely via the accessory pathway to the atria. Earliest atrial activation (A) is observed in the distal coronary sinus at electrodes 3,4 (CS 3,4). The wave of depolarization reengages the AV node and a reentrant circuit is initiated.

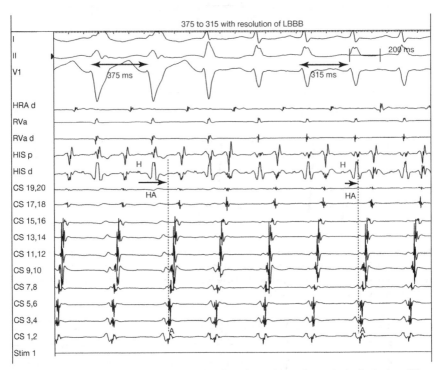

Figure 9.21 Resolution of left bundle branch block during tachycardia results in shortening of the tachycardia cycle length from 375 ms to 315 ms. This is mediated by significant shortening of the HA interval, which represents activation time from His depolarization to the first sign of atrial depolarization.

necessarily mean that the accessory pathway is involved in the tachycardia. For example, the patient may have an atrial tachycardia due to a focus within the left atrium, with the accessory pathway a "bystander." A comprehensive discussion of techniques for determining whether an accessory pathway is essential to the tachycardia circuit is beyond the scope of this introductory book, but the response of a tachycardia to bundle branch block can help provide some insight into thinking about tachycardias associated with accessory pathways.

Figure 9.21 shows the electrograms from a patient in tachycardia. Earliest atrial activation can be observed in the distal coronary sinus (A) at electrodes 3,4. Notice that with resolution of left bundle branch block the tachycardia cycle length decreases from 375 ms to 315 ms. The presence of this decrease in the tachycardia cycle length with resolution of left bundle branch block "proves" that the left bundle is a component of the tachycardia circuit and confirms the presence of a macroreentrant circuit that involves sequential activation of the accessory pathway, the left atrium, the AV node, and the left ventricle. A schematic of this phenomenon is shown in Fig. 9.22. The reader

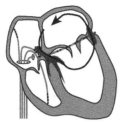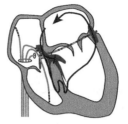

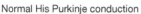
Normal His Purkinje conduction   Left bundle branch block

Figure 9.22 A schematic of the mechanism in Fig. 9.21. With resolution of left bundle branch block (normalization of the QRS width), the tachycardia cycle length shortens because the reentrant circuit can now utilize the left bundle.

can see that the shortening of the tachycardia cycle length is mainly due to shortening of the HA interval, which in this case represents the activation time within the ventricles. This finding is called Coumel's sign, in honor of the late Philippe Coumel, who described this response 40 years ago.

Ablation

The accessory pathway provides an ideal target for ablative therapy: a discrete anatomic site that once removed can "cure" a patient and eliminate symptoms. The location of the accessory pathway can be determined by either antero-grade mapping, looking for the earliest ventricular activation, or retrograde mapping, looking for the earliest site of atrial activation (Fig. 9.23).

An example of anterograde mapping is shown in Fig. 9.24. In patients with anterograde conduction, earliest ventricular activation is used to identify the ventricular insertion point of the accessory pathway. Sites on the annulus can be identified by moving the tip of the mapping catheter to sites with atrial and ventricular signals with equal amplitudes. Sites that are in the atria rather

Anterograde Mapping   Retrograde Mapping

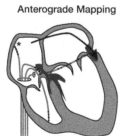

Earliest ventricular signal   Earliest atrial signal

Figure 9.23 Schematic of mapping techniques for localizing an accessory pathway. During sinus rhythm (anterograde mapping) the clinician "looks" for the earliest ventricular signal, and during retrograde mapping with ventricular pacing the clinician "looks" for the earliest atrial signal.

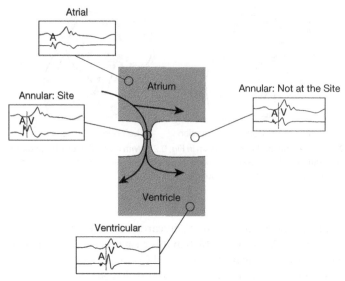

Figure 9.24 Schematic of anterograde mapping of the location of the accessory pathway during sinus rhythm. The catheter tip is moved to different sites. Annular sites can be identified by evaluating the relative sizes of the atrial (A) and ventricular (V) electrograms. If the catheter tip is at the annulus the atrial and ventricular electrograms will have similar amplitudes. Atrial locations will have larger atrial signals and ventricular sites will have larger ventricular signals. Once on the annulus, the site of the accessory pathway can be identified by locating the site with the earliest ventricular signal relative to the onset of the QRS complex.

than the annulus will have a larger atrial signal, and sites that are within the ventricle will have a larger ventricular signal. Along the annulus, the accessory pathway site will be identified by an early ventricular electrogram, which will in most cases precede the onset of the QRS complex. Ablation during sinus rhythm at a successful site is shown in Fig. 9.25. With application of radiofrequency energy, the QRS complex suddenly normalizes and an isoelectric PR interval is seen, signifying the loss of accessory pathway conduction (hopefully permanently).

Mapping can also be performed during ventricular pacing. An example of this mapping technique is shown in Fig. 9.26. During ventricular pacing, the catheter is carefully moved along annular sites until a site with the earliest atrial signal is identified. In the right panel of Fig. 9.26, during radiofrequency energy application, retrograde conduction via the accessory pathway is suddenly lost. The subsequent atrial activity is due to depolarization of the sinus node.

Finally, mapping can also be performed during supraventricular tachycardia. Since, during supraventricular tachycardia, depolarization is travelling retrogradely in the accessory pathway, the catheter is moved along the annulus to find the earliest atrial signal. An example of mapping and ablation during supraventricular tachycardia is shown in Fig. 9.27. During the ablation, the

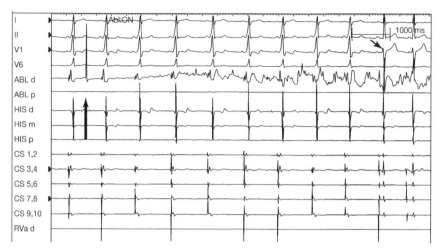

Figure 9.25 Ablation during sinus rhythm. After beginning ablation (large arrow), the QRS suddenly normalizes (small arrow) and an isoelectric PR interval can be observed when there is loss of accessory pathway conduction.

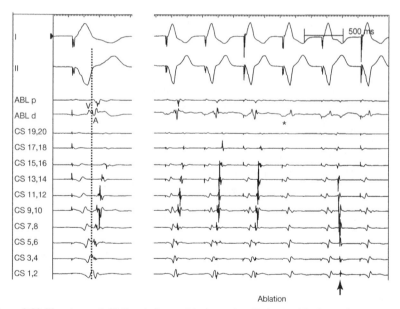

Ablation

Figure 9.26 Mapping and ablation during ventricular pacing. During ventricular pacing, the catheter tip is moved to an annular site with the earliest atrial signal. During ablation (right panel), there is sudden loss of retrograde accessory pathway conduction and 1 : 1 eccentric atrial activation (*). The subsequent atrial signal (arrow) is due to depolarization of the sinus node. A twenty-pole coronary sinus (CS) catheter has been inserted from the right internal jugular vein.

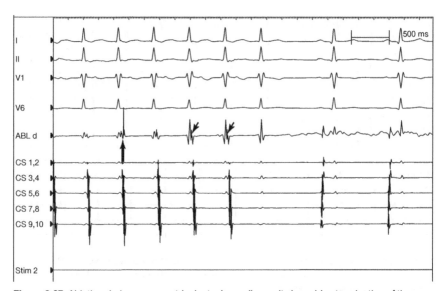

Figure 9.27 Ablation during supraventricular tachycardia results in sudden termination of the tachycardia quickly after starting the ablation (large arrow). A discrete pathway potential can be observed at the ablation site during ablation (small arrows).

tachycardia suddenly terminates when the accessory pathway is successfully ablated. One of the disadvantages of ablation during supraventricular tachycardia is that the sudden change in the ventricular rate can lead to catheter movement. To mitigate this effect, some clinicians will pace the heart at a rate slightly slower than the tachycardia rate, so that when the tachycardia terminates the ventricular rate remains unchanged. At this ablation site, a discrete "pathway potential" can be observed.

Regardless of the mapping approach, the ablation should be associated with loss of accessory pathway conduction within a short period of time (< 10 seconds). If loss of accessory pathway conduction occurs only after a prolonged period it is likely that accessory pathway conduction will return after time. In addidition, temperature should be carefully monitored during ablation. A site may be unsuccessful because of either inadequate localization or unstable catheter positioning.

After ablation, it is important to continue to evaluate the patient to determine whether accessory pathway conduction has recurred. Anterograde accessory conduction can be assessed by evaluating the QRS complex during sinus rhythm or atrial pacing. Ventricular pacing is used to determine whether retrograde conduction is present (Fig. 9.28).

The most common location for accessory pathways is the mitral annular free wall (> 50%), followed by septal sites (25–40%), with right atrial free-wall sites being the rarest (10–20%). Left-sided accessory pathways can be approached with a transseptal approach or retrograde through the aortic valve.

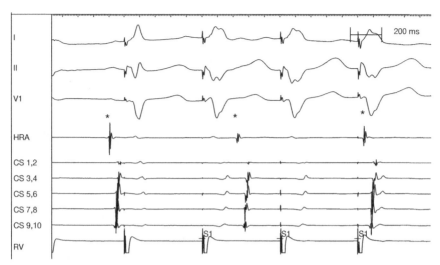

Figure 9.28 Absence of retrograde ventriculoatrial depolarization with ventricular pacing after successful ablation of an accessory pathway. During ventricular pacing, atrial activation is due to sinus rhythm, with earliest atrial activation (*) observed in the high right atrial (HRA) catheter.

Both techniques are effective, and choice often depends on patient preference. At our laboratory we prefer to use a transseptal approach for left-sided accessory pathways because of greater catheter stability on the mitral annulus. For right-sided and septal accessory pathways we find that long preshaped sheaths are helpful for stabilizing catheters on the tricuspid annulus.

Unusual accessory pathways

Most accessory pathways connect atrial and ventricular tissue and have normal conduction properties. However, accessory pathways with unusual characteristics or slow conduction have been identified. For example, in some cases an accessory pathway can connect from the specialized conducting tissue beyond the His bundle to ventricular tissue (Fig. 9.29). These fasciculoventricular

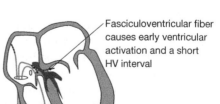

Fasciculoventricular fiber causes early ventricular activation and a short HV interval

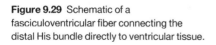

Figure 9.29 Schematic of a fasciculoventricular fiber connecting the distal His bundle directly to ventricular tissue.

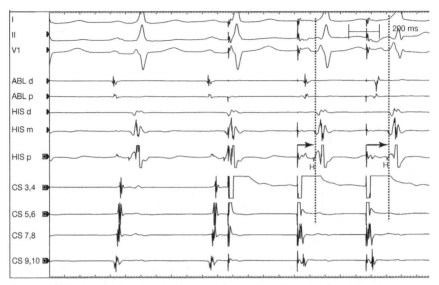

Figure 9.30 Atrial pacing in a patient with a fasciculoventricular fiber. Atrial pacing leads to a change in the QRS complex (because of more ventricular depolarization due to the fasciculoventricular fiber) but the HV interval remains constant even as the AH interval prolongs due to progressive slowing in AV nodal conduction (arrows).

connections can lead to abnormal-appearing QRS complexes because of abnormal ventricular depolarization and a very short HV interval, but they have not been implicated as a cause of tachycardia and are not associated with sudden cardiac death (since depolarization must still travel through the AV node. To take our earlier highway analogy one step further, one can imagine these accessory pathways as an "early additional" exit into the ventricle. An example of a fasciculoventricular fiber is shown in Fig. 9.30. The HV interval is very short, and with atrial pacing the QRS becomes wider. However, the short HV interval remains constant even with prolongation of the AH interval (arrows) and the onset of the QRS complex never occurs earlier than the His deflection.

In some very rare cases the accessory pathway will have slow conduction properties. A thorough discussion of these pathways is beyond the scope of this introductory text, but one example of an ablation of a slowly conducting accessory pathway is shown in Fig. 9.31. In this case the patient has a very slowly conducting accessory pathway near the coronary sinus os. Slow retrograde conduction leads to a very long interval between ventricular depolarization and the earliest atrial activation. Application of radiofrequency energy results in almost immediate termination of tachycardia. Histologic studies suggest that the slowly conducting proprerties of these pathways are due to their anatomic structure (long, thin, and serpiginous pathways) rather than

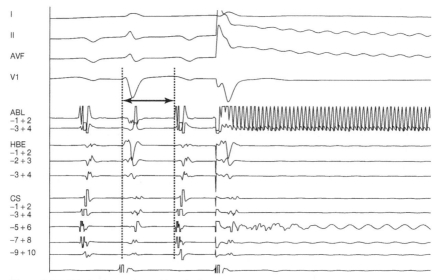

Figure 9.31 Ablation in a patient with a slowly conducting accessory pathway. The slow conduction properties of the accessory pathway lead to a very long ventriculoatrial conduction time (double-headed arrow) during supraventricular tachycardia. Earliest atrial activation occurs just within the coronary sinus (earliest at CS 5,6). With application of radiofrequency energy just within the os of the coronary sinus the tachycardia terminates almost immediately.

electrophysiologic properties (AV nodal-like tissue). This particular type of slowly conducting accessory pathway is sometimes called permanent junctional reciprocating tachycardia (PJRT, a name coined by Philippe Coumel), because the accessory pathways are near the AV node region and they are associated with incessant tachycardia.

CHAPTER 10

AV node reentry

Development of a reentrant circuit within the AV node or adjacent atrial tissue is the most common form of regular paroxysmal supraventricular tachycardia encountered in the electrophysiology laboratory. Reentry within the AV node was proposed in the early part of the twentieth century, first by Mines and soon afterwards by Iliescu and Sebastiani. The presence of dual/multiple inputs to the AV node as the substrate for reentry was described by a number of investigators in the 1960s and 1970s. In a large study of almost 2000 patients referred to the electrophysiology laboratory for supraventricular tachycardia, AV node reentry was the most commonly encountered arrhythmia: AV node reentry 56%; atrioventricular reentry using an accessory pathway 27%; atrial tachycardia 17%. Although accessory pathway-mediated tachycardia is more commonly encountered in children, by age 20 years AV node reentry becomes the dominant cause of paroxysmal regular tachycardia, particularly in women.

Anatomy and electrophysiology

In AV node reentry, the reentrant circuit is localized to regions within or adjacent to the AV node. The AV node is a complex structure, with the part known as the *compact AV node* located near the apex of the triangle of Koch. The triangle of Koch is an important landmark used by surgeons during valve surgeries to avoid injuring the AV node (Fig. 10.1). The triangle of Koch is bounded by the tricuspid valve and the tendon of Todaro on either side, with the base formed by the coronary sinus. There appear to be multiple extensions of cells with nodal properties that radiate from the compact AV node. It appears that these extensions form the substrate for the development of reentry by providing parallel, electrophysiologically separate pathways that meet at the compact AV node.

Although most likely a gross oversimplification of the true mechanism, AV node reentry is often considered as depending on two anatomically distinct pathways, with a "slow" pathway near the coronary sinus and a "fast" pathway superior to the triangle of Koch (Fig. 10.2). Although simplistic, this "working model" has provided the basis for much of our understanding and ablative approach to AV node reentry over the past two decades. In this model, during sinus rhythm conduction proceeds over the fast pathway (Fig. 10.3). In the most common form of AV node reentry, a premature atrial stimulus

Understanding Intracardiac EGMs and ECGs. By Fred Kusumoto. Published 2010 by Blackwell Publishing. ISBN: 978-1-4051-8410-6

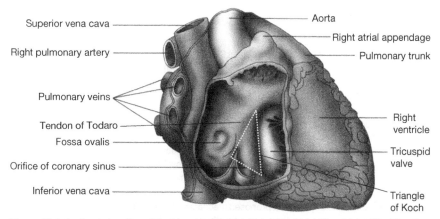

Figure 10.1 Anatomic location of the triangle of Koch in the right atrium. The sides of the triangle of Koch are defined by the tendon of Todaro and the tricuspid valve, with the base formed by the coronary sinus. (Adapted with permission from Kusumoto FM. Cardiovascular disorders: heart disease. In: McPhee SJ, Lingappa VR, Ganong WF, eds. *Pathophysiology of Disease*, 5th edn. New York, NY: McGraw-Hill, 2003.)

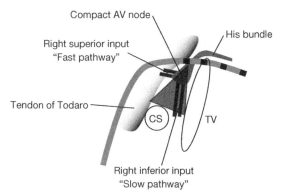

Figure 10.2 Schematic of the AV node. The compact AV node lies at the apex of the triangle of Koch (triangle bounded by dotted lines). The AV node has multiple "inputs" into the compact AV node, including a right superior input and a right inferior input. Generally, the right superior input has faster conduction properties than the right inferior input, so they are often called the "fast pathway" and the "slow pathway," respectively. CS, coronary sinus; TV, tricuspid valve.

blocks in the fast pathway and conducts slowly to the compact AV node via the "slow" pathway. If enough time has elapsed for the "fast" pathway to recover, a reentrant circuit will be initiated.

Electrocardiogram

At baseline, the ECG in patients with AV node reentry is often normal. Remember that depolarization of the AV node cannot be measured directly by intracardiac electrodes, so it is certainly not surprising that there are no specific findings on the ECG observed during sinus rhythm.

Sinus rhythm

Premature atrial contraction
initiates AVNRT

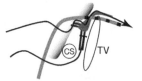 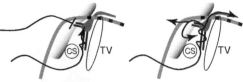

Normally conduction
through the "slow" pathway
is blocked due to
refractoriness in the AV node

Premature atrial contraction
blocks in the "fast" pathway but
conducts anterograde over the
"slow" pathway. If the "fast"
pathway has recovered, reentry
is initiated

Figure 10.3 Schematic showing the proposed mechanism for AV node reentry using a dual pathway model. During sinus rhythm conduction through the AV node proceeds over the "fast" pathway only. A premature atrial complex blocks in the "fast" pathway and conducts over the "slow" pathway. If the delay in the "slow" pathway is sufficient to allow recovery of the "fast" pathway the wave of depolarization can enter the "fast" pathway retrogradely and initiate AV node reentry. CS, coronary sinus; TV, tricuspid valve.

The ECG during supraventricular tachycardia can be very helpful for evaluating patients with AV node reentry. In the most common form of AV node reentry, P waves are often not observed during tachycardia because they are obscured by the larger QRS complex. The location of the P wave will depend on the relative conduction times of retrograde atrial depolarization and anterograde ventricular depolarization. In the "typical" form of AV node reentry, these times are almost equal, so atrial and ventricular depolarization are simultaneous. The P wave can sometimes be seen as a terminal negative deflection in the inferior leads and a terminal positive deflection in V_1. An ECG from a patient with AV node reentry is shown in Fig. 10.4. It is often very helpful to compare the QRS complexes during sinus rhythm and supraventricular tachycardia. Differences in the QRS morphology could be due to superimposed P waves. Figure 10.5 shows an ECG from the same patient in sinus rhythm. It can now be clearly seen that the small terminal positive deflection in lead V_1 was due to retrograde atrial depolarization.

Electrophysiologic findings

Electrophysiologic testing provides the "gold standard" for fully evaluating patients with AV node reentrant tachycardia. The presence of intracardiac electrograms allows definitive information on timing and spatial activation of the atria. The clinician can fully evaluate how the arrhythmia is initiated and terminated.

Atrial pacing

In the most common form of AV node reentry, premature atrial extrastimuli are delivered, and when a premature atrial extrastimulus encroaches on the

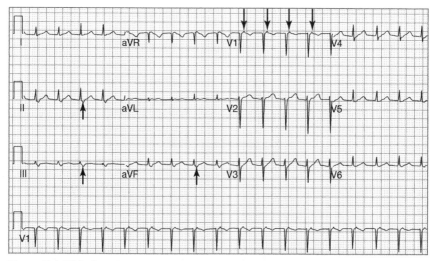

Figure 10.4 ECG of a patient with supraventricular tachycardia due to AV node reentry. Arrows show possible retrograde atrial activity present just after the QRS complex.

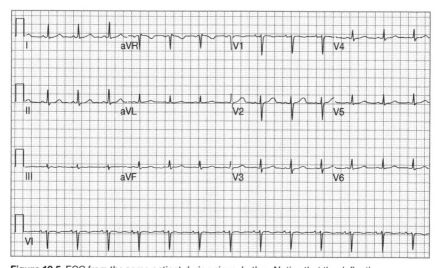

Figure 10.5 ECG from the same patient during sinus rhythm. Notice that the deflections associated with the arrows in Fig. 10.4 are no longer observed, confirming that the deflections most likely represent atrial depolarization.

refractory period of the fast pathway, sudden prolongation of the AH interval will be observed. In Fig. 10.6, a premature atrial stimulus is delivered at a coupling interval of 350 ms. As expected, there is prolongation of the AH interval due to decremental conduction within the AV node. In Fig. 10.7, the coupling interval is shortened to 340 ms. There is sudden prolongation of the AH interval because the "fast" pathway has blocked and conduction enters the

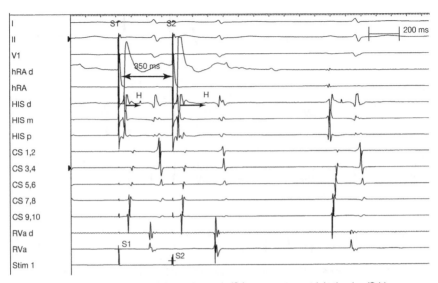

Figure 10.6 After a pacing train at 600 ms intervals (S_1), a premature atrial stimulus (S_2) is delivered at a coupling interval of 350 ms. As expected, the premature atrial stimulus is associated with a longer AH interval (arrow) due to decremental conduction within the AV node.

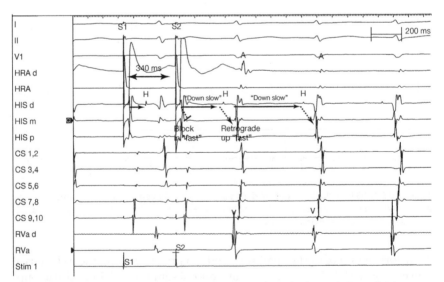

Figure 10.7 In the same patient as Fig. 10.6, the premature stimulus is coupled at a slightly shorter interval (340 ms). There is sudden prolongation of the AH interval and tachycardia is initiated. This finding is due to block in the "fast" pathway and conduction solely via the "slow" pathway. The slow conduction allows the "fast" pathway to recover, and AV node reentry is initiated.

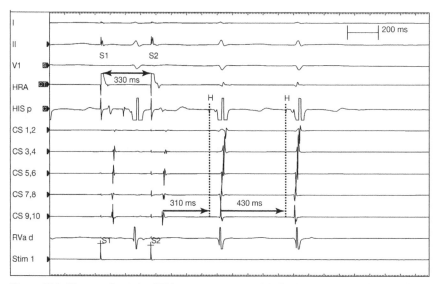

Figure 10.8 After a pacing train of 600 ms, a premature atrial stimulus at a coupling interval of 330 ms is delivered. This leads to two "echo" beats, but no sustained arrhythmia is induced, because of the development of block within the "slow" pathway.

AV node via the "slow" pathway. Slow conduction allows the "fast" pathway to recover and the wave of depolarization splits, one wave entering the "fast" pathway retrogradely and the other wave traveling normally over the His bundle to depolarize the ventricles. The "slow" pathway has recovered, and sustained AV node reentry is initiated.

At baseline in many cases, sustained AV node reentry is not initiated but "echo" beats can be seen. In Fig. 10.8, a premature atrial stimulus at a coupling interval of 330 ms is delivered, producing a QRS and an atrial depolarization (the depolarization has "echoed" back to the stimulation site), which in turn produces another echo beat. Notice that stable tachycardia is not produced because conduction in the "slow" pathway eventually blocks due to refractoriness. In this case sustained tachycardia is only produced when the "slow" pathway conduction is enhanced or "revved up," usually with the use of a beta-agonist such as isoproterenol. One can see why sustained AV node reentry is paroxysmal – it requires a perfectly timed premature beat in the setting of the proper sympathetic/parasympathetic input environment. This is also the reason that sometimes patients complain of supraventricular tachycardia only during exercise.

Ventricular pacing

Although it is more common to induce typical AV node reentry with atrial pacing, ventricular pacing can also initiate this arrhythmia. Figures 10.9 through 10.11 illustrate initiation of AV node reentrant tachycardia with ventricular pacing. In Fig. 10.9, pacing at a constant interval of 600 ms does

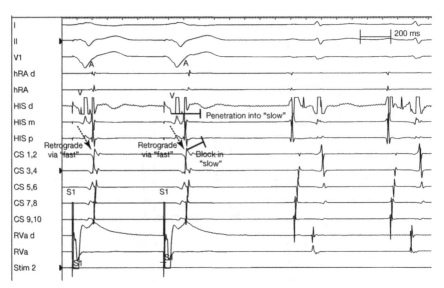

Figure 10.9 Ventricular pacing at a stimulus interval of 600 ms does not produce tachycardia on cessation of pacing.

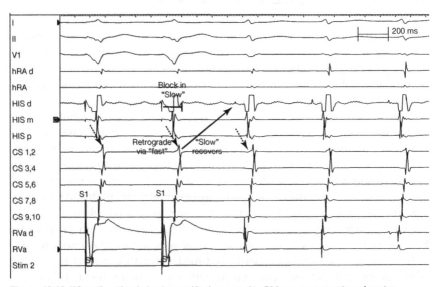

Figure 10.10 When the stimulation interval is decreased to 500 ms, on cessation of pacing, AV node reentry ensues.

not initiate tachycardia. However, when the pacing stimuli are delivered at 500 ms interval (Fig. 10.10), on cessation of pacing supraventricular tachycardia is initiated. Figure 10.11 illustrates the reason for the different response. At a stimulus interval of 600 ms, retrograde depolarization of both the "fast" and "slow" pathways is present. When the stimulus interval is decreased to

Ventricular pacing 600 ms   Ventricular pacing 500 ms

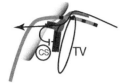   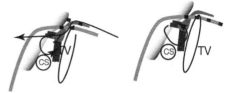

Retrograde penetration into   Retrograde block at the "entrance" of
the "slow" pathway prevents   the "slow" pathway allows
Initiation of reentry   anterograde conduction and initiation
                                                 of reentry

Figure 10.11 Schematic showing the reason for the different responses to the different stimulation intervals. At a 600 ms interval, retrograde conduction penetrates both the "fast" and "slow" pathways. When the interval is decreased to 500 ms, retrograde block in the "slow" pathway allows it to recover so the depolarization wave emerging from the "fast" pathway can split, with one wave reentering the "slow" pathway to initiate tachycardia. CS, coronary sinus; TV, tricuspid valve.

500 ms, retrograde block in the "slow" pathway develops, so that when pacing is stopped a reentrant tachycardia is initiated.

Tachycardia

In the typical form of AV node reentry, simultaneous atrial depolarization and ventricular depolarization is observed. As discussed in Chapter 5, the presence of nearly simultaneous ventricular and atrial activation rules out the use of an accessory pathway as the cause of tachycardia. Remember that in supraventricular tachycardia using an accessory pathway (orthodromic atrioventricular reentry) the atria and ventricles are depolarized sequentially, and a certain amount of time will be required to activate intervening ventricular tissue between the His–Purkinje system and the accessory pathway. The ventriculoatrial (VA) interval is used to measure the relationship between ventricular and atrial depolarization. The VA interval is usually measured from the initial QRS deflection to the first atrial electrogram (Fig. 10.12). In many cases the atrial component of the His bundle signal is obscured by the ventricular component, so the proximal coronary sinus at the os will often be the site of the first atrial depolarization in patients with AV node reentry. In an adult, a VA interval of less than 65 ms essentially rules out the presence of an accessory pathway.

When evaluating a supraventricular tachycardia with a VA interval < 65 ms the clinician must distinguish between AV node reentry and atrial tachycardia. Although this was covered in Chapter 5, it is worthwhile to review maneuvers to differentiate these two arrhythmias, since this problem is encountered very commonly in clinical practice (mainly because of the prevalence of AV node reentry in patients with supraventricular tachycardia). In atrial tachycardia, ventricular activation follows passively after atrial activity, so that when an atrial tachycardia site "stops" a subsequent ventricular depolarization will be observed. In AV node reentry, termination often occurs because of block in

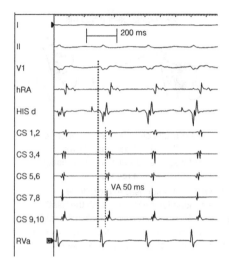

Figure 10.12 The VA interval is measured from the onset of the QRS complex to the earliest atrial signal (usually recorded in the coronary sinus os in patients with AV node reentry).

the "slow" pathway. As shown in Fig. 10.8, a tachycardia that "ends on an A," where the final signal is an atrial electrogram, rules out atrial tachycardia under most circumstances. Another technique is to deliver premature ventricular stimuli. If the tachycardia terminates without an atrial electrogram, it proves that the AV node is involved in the tachycardia (Fig. 10.13). If an atrial tachycardia was present the tachycardia would continue, since "it doesn't care about what is happening in the AV node." It is important for the clinician

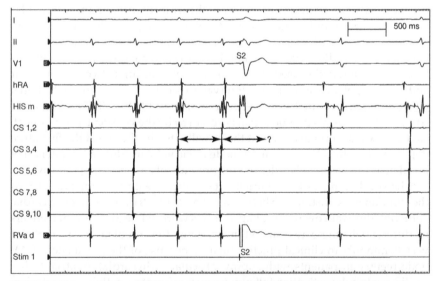

Figure 10.13 A premature ventricular stimulus (S$_2$) delivered during tachycardia terminates the supraventricular tachycardia. Termination occurred without an atrial electrogram (?). This finding proves that the AV node is involved in the tachycardia and rules out atrial tachycardia.

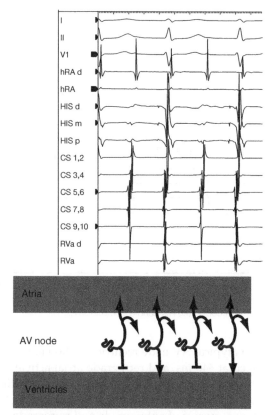

Figure 10.14 AV node reentry with 2 : 1 block to the ventricles. A schematic showing the tachycardia is shown below the electrograms for each beat. The patient has AV node reentrant tachycardia, retrograde activation of the atria occurs in a 1 : 1 fashion so that atrial electrograms are produced during each reentrant cycle. However, block in the AV node region proximal to the His bundle results in a 2 : 1 response for ventricular depolarization, and the ventricular rate is half the tachycardia rate.

not to be fooled by continuation of the tachycardia in the presence of AV block. In some cases AV node reentry will be associated with block in more distal portions of the atrioventricular conduction, leading to a 2 : 1 ventricular response (Fig. 10.14).

Although the most common form of AV node reentry involves anterograde conduction over the slow pathway and retrograde conduction over the fast pathway, the reader should intuitively realize that the typical pattern of AV node reentry is dependent on the relative conduction properties of the "slow" and "fast" pathways. In some cases, the tachycardia circuit can be reversed. Retrograde activation of the atria via the slow pathway will lead to a tachy-cardia with a long VA time. In a patient with two "slow" pathways, the VA time may be some intermediate value. Any of these forms of AV node reentry are grouped under the heading of *atypical AV node reentry*. In Fig. 10.15, electrograms

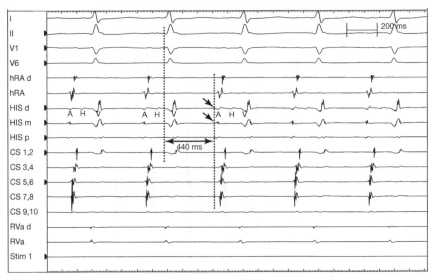

Figure 10.15 Electrograms from a patient with atypical AV node reentry. In this case retrograde activation occurs via the "slow" pathway, which leads to a very long VA interval. Earliest retrograde atrial activation occurs in the His bundle electrograms.

from a patient with atypical AV node reentry are shown. In this case the VA interval is prolonged at 440 ms, and retrograde atrial activation is occurring over a "slow" pathway. Earliest atrial activation is observed in the His catheter. AV node reentrant tachycardias are also commonly referred in "shorthand" by listing the activation sequence of anterograde and retrograde depolarization. Using this description, typical AV node reentry would be called "slow–fast," for anterograde activation via the "slow" pathway and retrograde activation via the "fast" pathway, and the atypical AV node reentrant tachycardias would be called "fast–slow" or "slow–slow." Using this nomenclature, the tachycardia shown in Fig. 10.15 would be classified as "fast–slow," since anterograde activation of the AV node (the AH interval) is normal.

Ablation

Ablation techniques for AV node reentry were first developed in the late 1980s. Originally the fast pathway was targeted, but because of an unacceptable rate of AV block, today radiofrequency catheter ablation techniques are designed to target the "slow" pathway (Fig. 10.16). Normally the "slow" pathway is located in tissue just anterior to the coronary sinus. Fluoroscopy from a patient undergoing radiofrequency catheter ablation of the slow pathway is shown in Fig. 10.17. The ablation catheter is located at the level of the coronary sinus catheter and positioned closer to the tricuspid valve. The characteristics of electrograms at successful sites have been described by a number of investigators. The tricuspid valve is more apically displaced than the mitral valve. For this reason when on the right atrial septal wall near the tricuspid

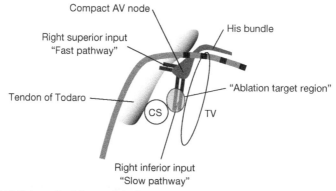

Figure 10.16 Schematic of the usual site for ablation of AV node reentry attempting to target the "slow" pathway. CS, coronary sinus; TV, tricuspid valve.

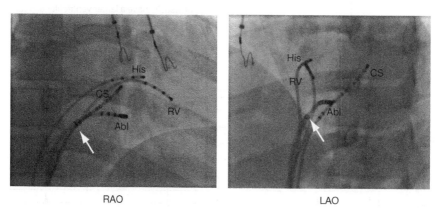

Figure 10.17 Fluoroscopic images in the right anterior oblique (RAO) and left anterior oblique (LAO) projections. The coronary sinus (CS) and His catheters are used to provide landmarks for the superior and inferior limits of the Triangle of Koch. A long sheath (arrow) is used to stabilize the ablation (Abl) catheter tip.

valve a large ventricular electrogram is recorded because of the underlying left ventricular septum. The atrial signal often is complex, and in some cases a discrete potential will be observed. Two examples of electrograms from successful ablation sites are shown in Fig. 10.18.

With application of ablation energy, junctional rhythm may be observed, although this is a nonspecific finding. The junctional rhythm appears to be due to increased automaticity and heat sensitivity of this tissue. Figure 10.19 shows development of junctional rhythm with application of radiofrequency energy.

Given the proximity of the ablation site to the AV node, it is critical to continuously monitor the electrograms and ECG during ablation to reduce the risk of heart block. When junctional rhythm occurs there should be retrograde fast pathway conduction. If a junctional beat is noted without an accompanying retrograde atrial electrogram, energy application should be stopped immediately. In addition, any prolongation of the AH interval during ablation or dropped QRS (isolated atrial electrogram or P wave without a subsequent

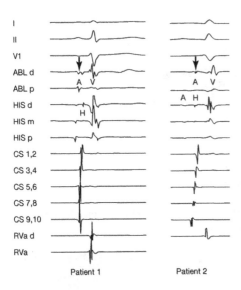

Figure 10.18 Electrograms from successful ablation sites for "slow" pathway modification. The electrograms will usually have a larger ventricular signal, and the atrial signal will often have a complex fractionated appearance (arrows).

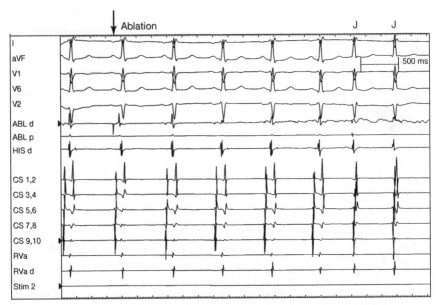

Figure 10.19 Development of junctional beats (J) after starting ablation. Junctional beats can be identified by initial His bundle signal and will often have an atrial electrogram observed at the same time as the QRS complex, due to retrograde conduction via the "fast" pathway.

QRS) should signal stopping application of ablation. It is critical to stop radiofrequency energy quickly once any evidence for injury to AV nodal conduction is identified, to reduce the likelihood of permanent damage to atrioventricular conduction, and it is important to remember that AV nodal block can occur in almost any region in the triangle of Koch. Figure 10.20

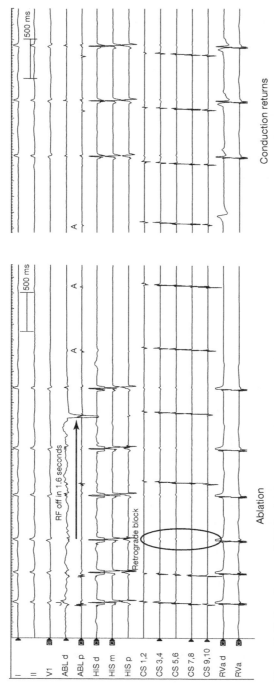

Ablation

Conduction returns

Figure 10.20 Development of AV block during an ablation procedure. The ablation catheter tip is located in a region close to the inferior portion of the coronary sinus greater than 2 cm from a previously recorded His signal. Radiofrequency energy results in junctional rhythm (J), but abruptly retrograde block in the fast pathway occurs (QRS without an accompanying atrial electrogram). Despite stopping the ablation within two seconds, high-grade AV block occurs, with nonconducted atrial depolarization (A). Fortunately, within a minute, AV conduction returns.

shows a sequence of electrograms recorded during and after ablation at a region located 2 cm away from the His catheter. After eight seconds of ablation, junctional rhythm is noted, but the patient develops an early junctional beat and abruptly retrograde block in the fast pathway is noted by the junctional beat without an accompanying atrial electrogram. Even after stopping radiofrequency energy within two seconds of the first sign of fast pathway

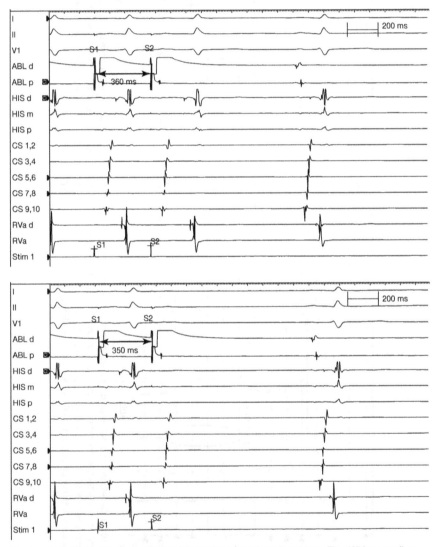

Figure 10.21 End point after a successful ablation of the "slow" pathway. *Top*: With a coupling interval of 360 ms, AV conduction occurs via the "fast" pathway. *Bottom:* When the coupling interval is decreased to 350 ms the AV node effective refractory period is reached, and instead of "switching to slow," atrial depolarization simply blocks in the "fast" pathway.

block, complete AV block is initially observed. Fortunately, within a minute, normal atrioventricular conduction returns. Because of the proximity to the AV node, some clinicians will use cryoablation energy at these sites, particularly in children.

Once ablation is performed, the patient should be evaluated for inducibility of AV node reentry. Oftentimes if the "slow" pathway has been ablated the response shown in Fig. 10.21 will be observed. In this example, when the premature atrial stimulus is coupled earlier, when block in the "fast" pathway develops, since there is no "slow" pathway for the depolarization to "switch" to, AV node block is observed. It does appear that one simply has to "modify" the AV node, and that the presence of a single echo beat when the patient had inducible sustained AV node reentry prior to the ablation is a satisfactory end point.

CHAPTER 11

Focal atrial tachycardia

There are a number of different types of arrhythmias that arise from atrial tissue. The following three chapters will discuss electrophysiologic testing and ablation techniques in patients with focal atrial tachycardia, atrial flutter, and atrial fibrillation. Tachycardias due to rapid but regular atrial activation are classified as *atrial flutter* or *focal atrial tachycardia*. Atrial flutter is characterized by a large macroreentrant circuit within the atria, while focal atrial tachycardia is due to a point source, regardless of mechanism – abnormal automaticity, triggered activity, or microreentry. Although this distinction is somewhat arbitrary (how large is large?) it is clinically useful, since it helps plan ablation strategy – ablation of a focal source versus ablation across a critical isthmus. In this chapter electrophysiology and ablation of focal atrial tachycardia will be discussed.

Electrophysiology and anatomy

Focal atrial tachycardias are uncommon, with an overall prevalence of less than 0.5%. They are the least common type of paroxysmal supraventricular tachycardia found at electrophysiologic testing, accounting for less than 10% of cases in large series. Mechanistically, abnormal automaticity is the most common cause of atrial tachycardia, particularly in children. Arrhythmias due to triggered activity can also be seen in children. Small reentrant circuits appear to be a more common cause of focal atrial tachycardia in adults. Adenosine is sometimes used to identify the putative mechanism for an atrial tachycardia. Adenosine will cause abrupt termination of arrhythmias due to triggered activity (adenosine-sensitive) and reentry, while abnormal automaticity will be transiently suppressed without termination. However, studies that systematically evaluated adenosine have yielded mixed results. Regardless of mechanism, focal atrial tachycardias appear to arise from specific sites, and often the surface ECG P wave and endocardial activation pattern will give the clinician some direction for identifying the source of the arrhythmia.

In the right atrium the most common site for atrial tachycardia is the crista terminalis, which is a long ridge that travels vertically along the anterior and lateral right atrium. Other less common right atrial sites for atrial tachycardia

Understanding Intracardiac EGMs and ECGs. By Fred Kusumoto. Published 2010 by Blackwell Publishing. ISBN: 978-1-4051-8410-6

foci include the right atrial appendage, the tricuspid annulus, the coronary sinus os, and within the triangle of Koch.

In the left atrium the most common site are the pulmonary veins. Analogous to the right atrium, focal tachycardias from the left atrial appendage, the mitral annulus, and the left atrial side of the septum, particularly near Bachmann's bundle, have also been reported.

Electrocardiogram

The morphology of the P wave can provide clues to the location of the atrial tachycardia. Unfortunately, P waves can be small and at times are obscured by the T wave from the preceding QRS complex. Sometimes infusion with adenosine can be helpful for providing "unadulterated" P waves by producing ventricular asystole (Fig. 11.1). Focal atrial tachycardias will generally have a discrete baseline separating atrial depolarizations, while macroreentrant circuits associated with atrial flutter will sometimes have no true isoelectric phase (Fig. 11.2). Since, even with macroreentrant circuits, regions of the flutter circuit can sometimes be "electrocardiographically silent," the author has found that the absence of a true isoelectric period is helpful for identifying atrial flutter, but the presence of an isoelectric period is less helpful.

The morphology of the P wave can provide useful clues for identifying the location of the atrial tachycardia (Table 11.1). However, it is important to acknowledge the limitations of examining P wave morphology, particularly given their small size and that their true shape is often obscured by the QRS complex or T waves. In one study, sites separated by 2–3 cm yielded P waves of identical morphology.

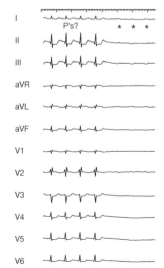

Figure 11.1 ECG from a patient with atrial tachycardia. It is difficult to determine the shape and number of P waves, because of the QRS complex and the T wave. Infusion with adenosine allows easier evaluation of the P wave morphology. In this case the positive P wave in aVL suggests that the focal atrial tachycardia is in the right atrium.

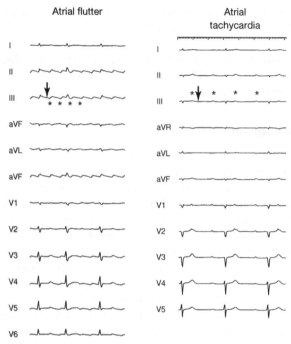

Figure 11.2 ECGs from atrial flutter and atrial tachycardia. Since atrial flutter may involve a large macroreentrant circuit, flutter waves (*) are not separated by a true isoelectric period (arrow). In contrast, in focal atrial tachycardias, a true isoelectric period with no evidence of atrial activation will be seen.

Table 11.1 ECG clues for locating the site of atrial tachycardia.

Location	ECG characteristics
Right atrium	
Crista terminalis	Negative in aVR
	Biphasic (positive then negative) in V_1
Coronary sinus os	Positive in aVL
	Negative in II, III, and aVF
Left atrium	
Pulmonary veins	Positive in V_1–V_6
Mitral annulus	Biphasic P wave (negative then positive) in V_1
	Low amplitude waves in the frontal leads

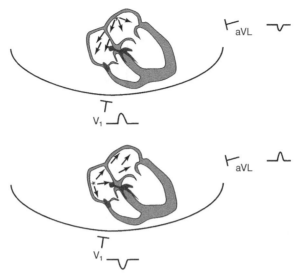

Figure 11.3 Schematic showing ECG criteria for determining whether a patient has a right atrial or left atrial tachycardia.

Clinically, it is important to determine whether an atrial tachycardia is arising from the left atrium or the right atrium on the surface ECG. Historically, this distinction was very important because of the additional morbidity associated with left atrial access and transseptal puncture. Although new technologies have made left atrial access simpler and safer, it is always important for the clinician to make a "best guess" as to whether the tachycardia focus is in the left or right atrium. The best leads to make this distinction are leads V_1 and aVL. An upright P wave in lead V_1 is very suggestive of a left atrial focus, with a positive predictive value of almost 90%. This association is due to the more posterior location of the left atrium and the resulting posterior-to-anterior activation direction. In contrast, a positive P wave in aVL is very suggestive of a right atrial focus, with a positive predictive value of approximately 80% (Fig. 11.3). It is important to evaluate P wave morphology even if the atrial rate appears normal. Figure 11.4 shows a patient referred for "sinus tachycardia" and chronic tiredness. However, notice that the P wave is inverted in aVL and positive in aVR and V_1. At electrophysiology study a left atrial tachycardia focus from the lateral wall of the left atrium was identified. After ablation, the ECG in Fig. 11.5 was recorded and the patient no longer complained of fatigue and shortness of breath.

Electrophysiology

Atrial tachycardias can sometimes be initiated with rapid atrial pacing or with premature atrial extrastimuli in patients with microreentrant citcuits.

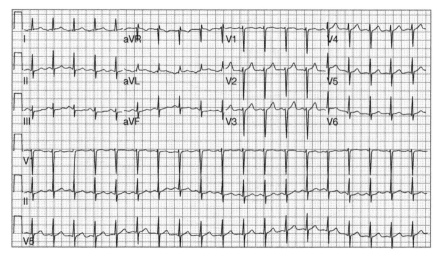

Figure 11.4 ECG from a patient referred for resting "sinus tachycardia." Notice that the P wave is inverted in lead aVL and upright in aVR. In a patient with sinus rhythm the P wave should be negative in aVR and positive in aVL. At electrophysiology study the patient was found to have an incessant focal atrial tachycardia from the left atrium. (Reprinted with permission from Kusumoto FM. *ECG Interpretation: From Pathophysiology to Clinical Application*. New York, NY: Springer, 2009.)

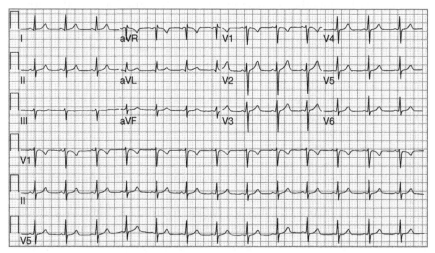

Figure 11.5 ECG from the same patient as Fig. 11.4 after successful ablation. Notice that the P waves now have a normal morphology. (Reprinted with permission from Kusumoto FM. *ECG Interpretation: From Pathophysiology to Clinical Application*. New York, NY: Springer, 2009.)

Figure 11.6 shows an atrial tachycardia induced with a premature atrial stimulus. At a coupling interval of 510 ms an atrial tachycardia is initiated. Notice that the atrial tachycardia is associated with 2:1 atrioventricular conduction. Unfortunately, if the atrial tachycardia is due to abnormal

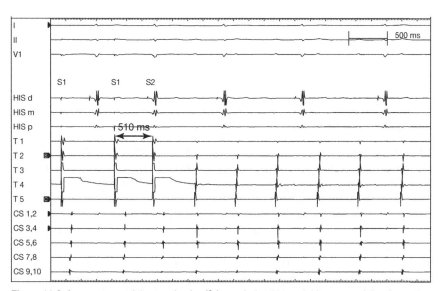

Figure 11.6 A premature atrial extrastimulus (S₂) coupled at 510 ms initiates an atrial tachycardia. A decapolar catheter has been placed along the lateral wall of the right atrium (T1–T5). CS, coronary sinus; His, His bundle.

automaticity, programmed extrastimuli are often ineffective for initiating tachycardia. In most cases, isoproterenol (or less frequently caffeine or theophylline) is required to initiate the tachycardia. Similarly, once initiated, most atrial tachycardias will terminate spontaneously. However, there are exceptions.

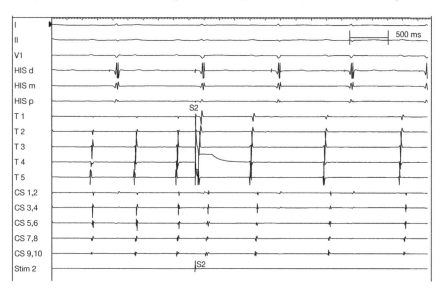

Figure 11.7 The same patient as Fig. 11.6. During atrial tachycardia, a single premature atrial extrastimulus (S₂) terminates the tachycardia. Initiation and termination of any tachycardia with premature extrastimuli suggests reentry as the underlying mechanism. Abbreviations as in Fig. 11.6.

In Fig. 11.7, the same patient shown in Fig. 11.6 has termination of his atrial tachycardia with a single premature atrial extrastimulus. Initiation or termination of tachycardia with premature atrial extrastimuli suggest that microreentry is the mechanism for an atrial tachycardia, although in some cases triggered activity can also display this response.

Mapping and ablation

Once initiated, focal atrial tachycardias are methodically mapped to identify the source of the tachycardia. In general, the strategy for mapping involves first identifying a "region of interest" and then using multipolar catheters within that region to identify the specific point source of the focal atrial tachycardia.

Usually evaluation of the P wave on surface ECG and evaluation of the timing and pattern of electrograms in the coronary sinus and the right atrium will provide a general guide for the location: right atrium versus left atrium, high versus low, back versus front. An example of the process of mapping atrial tachycardia in a single patient is shown in Figs. 11.8 through 11.12.

Figure 11.8 shows an irregular tachycardia that was interpreted as atrial fibrillation. Figure 11.9 shows the electrograms during tachycardia. It is now apparent that a regular atrial tachycardia is present and that the irregular ventricular rate was due to changes in AV conduction. Inspection of the electrograms provides important information for the general location of the atrial tachycardia. First, it appears that the left atrium (as represented by the atrial signals in the coronary sinus catheter) and the right atrium (as represented by a decapolar catheter placed in the superior and lateral wall of the right atrium with the tip pointed down) are being activated at the same time. Figures 11.10

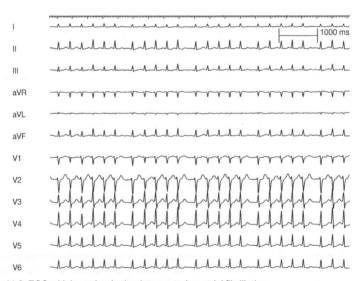

Figure 11.8 ECG with irregular rhythm interpreted as atrial fibrillation.

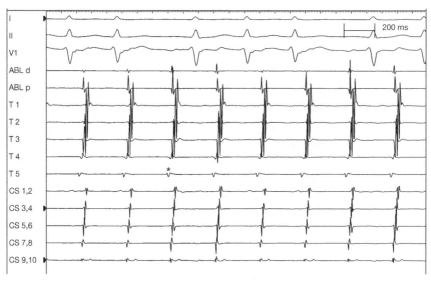

Figure 11.9 Intracardiac electrograms from the patient in Fig. 11.8. It is now evident that regular atrial depolarization is present, and that the irregular ventricular rhythm is due to changing AV conduction. In this patient a mobile mapping catheter (ABL) is located at the superior vena cava–right atrial junction, a decapolar catheter is placed along the lateral wall of the right atrium with the catheter tip pointed downward (T1–T5), and a decapolar catheter is in the coronary sinus. The earliest atrial electrogram (*) is noted in the most proximal electrode pair in the catheter placed in the lateral right atrium (T5).

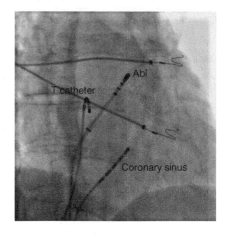

Figure 11.10 Right anterior oblique (RAO) fluoroscopic view of typical catheter positions for mapping atrial tachycardias. A decapolar catheter is placed in the coronary sinus and a second decapolar catheter is placed in the superior and lateral wall of the right atrium (T catheter). A roving catheter for mapping and ablation (Abl) is also shown. The ablation catheter in this fluoroscopy image is placed anteriorly and septally within the left atrium. Electrograms from this site are shown in Fig. 11.13.

and 11.11 show fluoroscopic images of the decapolar catheters located in the right atrium and coronary sinus. Earliest atrial electrical activity appears to be in the superior portion of the right atrium along the interatrial septum at T5 (designated by the asterisk in Fig. 11.9). However, when the gain is increased

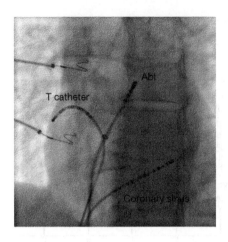

Figure 11.11 Left anterior oblique (LAO) fluoroscopic view of the catheters from Fig. 11.10. This angle shows that the T catheter is located along the superior and lateral walls of the right atrium and the mapping/ablation catheter (Abl) is located on the septal side of the left atrium.

in surface ECG lead V_1, it is evident that the electrogram recorded from T5 is actually not very early, suggesting that all of the electrodes are located "far away" from the tachycardia site (Fig. 11.12). In addition, increasing the gain on lead V_1 reveals a biphasic P wave with initial negative and terminal positive deflections. The area that is not evaluated by this catheter configuration is the superior and posterior left atrium. Reviewing Table 11.1, this P wave morphology is more consistent with a site near the mitral annulus rather than

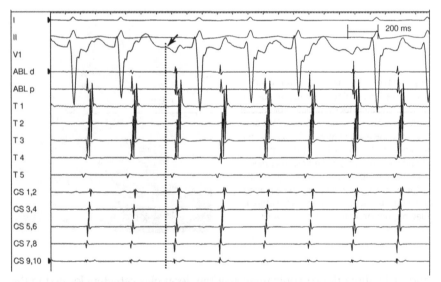

Figure 11.12 Utility of changing the gain for identifying the relative positions of electrograms. Notice that when the gain in lead V_1 is increased the downstroke of the P wave (arrow) can be seen, and it is evident that all of the electrograms are late relative to the onset of the P wave (dotted vertical line). Abbreviations as in Fig. 11.9.

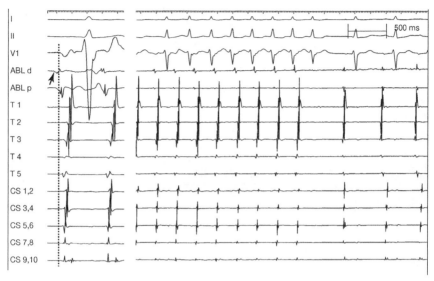

Figure 11.13 The left atrium was entered via transseptal access. The left atrium was mapped extensively, and at a septal site in the left atrium near the mitral annulus (shown in Figs. 11.10 and 11.11) a site with an atrial electrogram that preceded the P wave was found (arrow). With application of radiofrequency energy, the atrial tachycardia terminated within 2 seconds.

near the pulmonary veins (in which a positive P wave would be expected). Transseptal access was performed and regions in the left atrium were mapped. Electrograms from the site shown in Figs. 11.10 and 11.11 are shown in Fig. 11.13. Notice that at this superior septal site near the mitral annulus the atrial electrogram precedes the onset of the P wave. Radiofrequency energy application here resulted in prompt termination of the atrial tachycardia. This case illustrates the standard method for mapping atrial tachycardia. Since one is searching for a point source, a mapping catheter is moved methodically to search for an electrogram that occurs early relative to a fixed point. If possible, a point on the surface P wave should be used as a reference point, although an intracardiac catheter with a stable position (usually the coronary sinus catheter) can also be used. The surface P wave is generally preferable, but sometimes the onset can be difficult to identify.

Sometimes multipolar catheters with complex designs can be useful for quickly identifying atrial tachycardia sites. Figure 11.14 shows a right anterior oblique image of a multipolar basket catheter placed in the right upper pulmonary vein. Electrograms from the basket catheter are shown in Fig. 11.15. The earliest atrial signal arises from electrodes 3,4 on the G spline (marked in Figs. 11.14 and 11.15 with an asterisk). Atrial tachycardia from within the pulmonary vein depolarizes the rest of the pulmonary vein and the rest of the atrium. Unfortunately, sites within the pulmonary vein are not amenable to ablation because of the possibility of scar tissue formation at the ablation site causing pulmonary vein stenosis. In this case, a series of ablations are

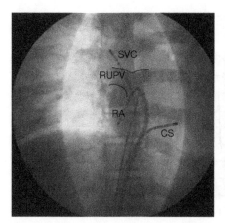 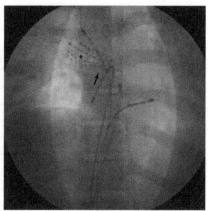

Figure 11.14 *Left*: Angiogram of the left atrium and the right upper pulmonary vein (RUPV). Decapolar catheters are located in the superior vena cava (SVC), coronary sinus (CS), and right atrium (RA). *Right:* A multipolar basket catheter is placed in the right upper pulmonary vein. Asterisk (*) marks site of earliest electrical signal. The arrow marks the position of the right upper pulmonary vein ostium.

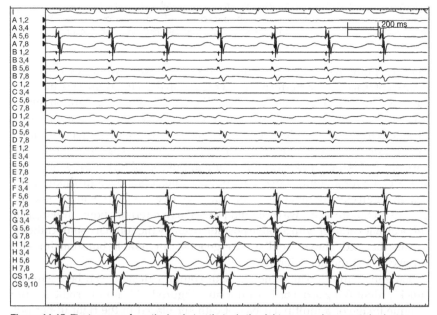

Figure 11.15 Electrograms from the basket catheter in the right upper pulmonary vein shown in Fig. 11.14. The earliest atrial signal is at electrode pair 3,4 in the G spline (* in Figs. 11.14 and 11.15). Letters A–H identify the splines of the basket catheter, with the more proximal electrode pairs numbered 5,6 and 7,8; CS, coronary sinus electrodes.

performed just outside the pulmonary vein in an attempt to isolate the vein from the left atrium. In Fig. 11.16, as the circumferential ablation is completed, the atrial tachycardia terminates. When the basket catheter is reinserted into the pulmonary vein (Fig. 11.17) it is obvious that the atrial tachycardia in the

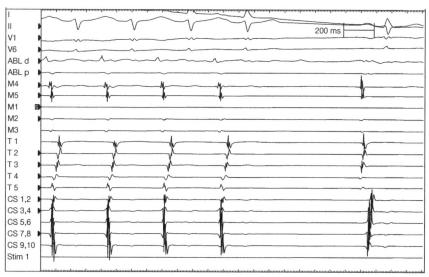

Figure 11.16 As ablation is performed in the left atrium around the right upper pulmonary vein, the tachycardia "terminates." ABL, ablation catheter; M1–M5, decapolar catheter placed in the left atrium; T1–T5, decapolar catheter in the right atrium; CS, coronary sinus.

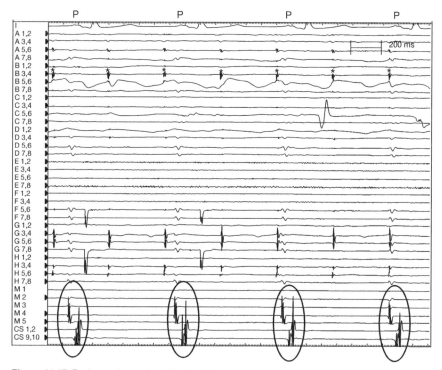

Figure 11.17 Basket catheter placed in the right upper pulmonary vein (it was removed during ablation) reveals continued atrial tachycardia in the pulmonary vein (*). However, depolarization is blocked and does not conduct to the atria. Independent P waves and right and left atrial depolarization (ellipses) can be seen. Letters A–H identify the splines of the basket catheter, with the more proximal electrode pairs numbered 5,6 and 7,8; CS, coronary sinus electrodes.

pulmonary vein continues, but conduction from the pulmonary veins is blocked and the atria are depolarized by the sinus node.

Advanced mapping systems provide important supplemental information for identifying the critical site for ablation. In fact, three-dimensional mapping systems have revolutionized ablation for atrial tachycardia. However, understanding the fundamental electrophysiologic principles is an essential first step for understanding more complex ablation procedures.

CHAPTER 12

Atrial flutter

Traditionally, atrial flutter has been defined as abnormally rapid organized atrial activity identified by the 12-lead ECG. More recently, with the elucidation of the reentrant circuit in typical atrial flutter, from an electrophysiologic standpoint the term *atrial flutter* is used to define abnormal atrial activity due to a reentrant circuit, while *focal atrial tachycardia* is used to describe abnormal atrial activity due to a "point source" such as a nest of cells with abnormal automaticity. As pointed out in the previous chapter this is an imperfect definition, since a very small microreentrant circuit can appear to be a point source during electrophysiologic testing. However, it is a clinically useful approach in the electrophysiology laboratory since it dictates the most effective ablation strategy. The main issue is whether to ablate a single "earliest" site, as discussed in the last chapter for ablation of focal atrial tachycardia, or to define critical channels defined by scars that should be ablated by creating a line of block across the scar (Fig. 12.1). Table 12.1 summarizes the important clinical questions for evaluating abnormally rapid atrial activity, and atrial flutter in particular – What is the mechanism of the tachycardia? Is the reentrant circuit large (macroreentrant) or small? Is the critical portion of the circuit in the right or left atrium? What structures/scars may be contributing to the formation of a "critical isthmus?"

Mechanism

Since the definition of atrial flutter depends so much on mechanism, once a rapid atrial arrhythmia is induced the clinician will need to characterize the mechanism of a tachycardia. If available, inspection of spontaneous initiation and termination should be evaluated. Atrial tachycardias due to automaticity just "start," whereas reentrant arrhythmias are initiated by a premature beat that is usually different from the tachycardia itself (P waves will be different, endocardial electrograms will be different). The characteristics of spontaneous termination are less helpful, but termination with a single premature beat makes reentry much more likely.

Instead of depending on spontaneous initiation and termination, during electrophysiologic testing the clinician can artificially introduce extrastimuli to

Understanding Intracardiac EGMs and ECGs. By Fred Kusumoto. Published 2010 by Blackwell Publishing. ISBN: 978-1-4051-8410-6

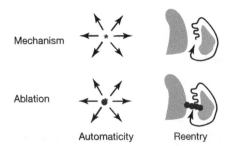

Figure 12.1 Ablation strategy based on mechanism. In an arrhythmia due to abnormal automaticity, ablation is performed by locating the earliest electrogram and ablating at that point source. In a patient with reentry (often using fixed scars or barriers such as the tricuspid valve or venous entry points), ablation is performed by determining the critical channel(s) used by the reentrant circuit and creating an ablation line across the channel that prevents conduction and utilization of the channel for reentry.

Table 12.1 Important issues for evaluation and treatment of atrial flutter in the electrophysiology laboratory.

Questions	Specific points
Reentrant or focal?	Initiation with premature atrial contractions suggests reentry. Initiation with overdrive atrial pacing and isoproterenol can be seen with both mechanisms. Spontaneous initiation of the tachycardia suggests automaticity
	Termination with premature atrial contractions suggest reentry
	Evidence for entrainment: progressive fusion suggests reentry
	"Late meets early" suggests reentry
Size of the reentrant circuit?	Large circuits will tend to have atrial signals observed through the entire cycle length
Left or right atrium?	Shorter return cycle lengths will be observed during entrainment mapping as the pacing site is moved closer and closer to the reentrant circuit
Where is the critical isthmus?	What electrograms are recorded during the "isoelectric" period between flutter waves?
	Pacing from a site that demonstrates "concealed" entrainment

initiate or terminate arrhythmias. Traditionally, the ability to initiate a tachy-cardia with premature stimuli or pace-terminate a tachycardia has been used as the sine qua non for the existence of a reentrant mechanism. However, it has been known for over 30 years that arrhythmias due to triggered activity (a form of abnormal automaticity) can also be terminated by rapid pacing. The response of the tachycardia to different slightly faster pacing rates can identify the presence of entrainment. Entrainment will be discussed more fully in the discussion of typical atrial flutter, but the reader should understand that the presence of entrainment is an important clue for confirming an underlying reentrant mechanism.

Response to drugs can also be useful for differentiating arrhythmia mechanism. In a patient with the tachycardia isolated to atrial tissue (AV node-independent) adenosine will generally not affect a tachycardia that is due to a macroreentrant mechanism, although it may terminate arrhythmias due to triggered activity and arrhythmias due to "microreentry."

Cavotricuspid isthmus-dependent atrial flutter

The most commonly observed atrial flutters use the isthmus formed by the inferior vena cava and the tricuspid valve as the critical region of "protected" slow conduction. In "typical" atrial flutter, the wave of atrial depolarization travels from the lateral right atrium, through the isthmus to the inferior portion of the interatrial septum. The wave of depolarization splits and travels in the inferior–superior direction in the interatrial septum and the lateral wall of the left atrium. The circuit is completed as the wave of depolarization travels around the tricuspid valve to reactivate the lateral wall of the right atrium. This typical pattern will lead to flutter waves that are negative in the inferior leads (II, III, and aVF) although there will be significant variability. The specific ECG pattern of the flutter waves can be quite variable, with no specific correlates for baseline P waves during sinus rhythm or echocardiographic manifestations of left atrial size or shape. Careful simultaneous inspection of the flutter waves will reveal that often there is no truly isoelectric period (Fig. 12.2).

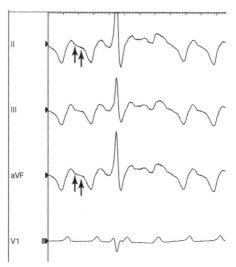

Figure 12.2 Rhythm strip from a patient with typical atrial flutter with increased gains. Notice that in the inferior leads there is no true isoelectric period between flutter waves (arrows).

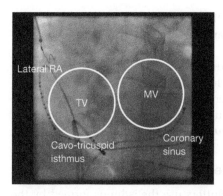

Figure 12.3 Fluoroscopic image in the left anterior oblique (LAO) projection of a commonly used catheter set. In this case a multipolar catheter is placed in the coronary sinus to provide signals from the left atrium, a multipolar catheter is placed in the lateral wall of the right atrium (RA), and a large-tipped ablation catheter is placed within the cavotricuspid isthmus. MV, mitral valve; TV, tricuspid valve.

Since the cavotricuspid isthmus is such a common site for the critical isthmus for most clinically encountered atrial flutters, the first step in the electrophysiologic evaluation of atrial flutter is to determine whether the arrhythmia is isthmus-dependent.

Reference catheters are placed in positions that can record signals from both atria. Usually a multipolar catheter is placed in the coronary sinus to record left atrial activity and another multipolar catheter is placed in the lateral wall of the right atrium. Finally, a mapping catheter is placed in the cavotricuspid isthmus (Fig. 12.3). Baseline electrograms are shown in Fig. 12.4. In typical atrial flutter, atrial activation proceeds from superior to inferior along the lateral wall of the right atrium, travels through the cavotricuspid isthmus, and then travels from inferior to superior along the course of the coronary sinus in the left atrium. At the same time as the coronary sinus region of the left atrium is being activated, atrial activation travels in the inferior-to-superior direction along the interatrial septum. In typical atrial flutter the signal from the cavotricuspid isthmus occurs just before the coronary sinus. Notice also that since this is a macroreentrant circuit, "continuous" atrial electrograms can be observed in large regions of the heart. The electrograms also illustrate that the negative portion of the flutter wave in the inferior leads is due to inferior-to-superior activation of the interatrial septum and the left atrium.

To test whether the cavotricuspid isthmus is the critical region of conduction, pacing maneuvers called *entrainment mapping* are performed in this region. Entrainment mapping techniques are an essential part of the electrophysiologic evaluation of any reentrant arrhythmia, but are particularly useful for identifying the location of reentrant circuits within the atria or the ventricles. A useful analogy for entrainment mapping is to think of a reentrant circuit as a circulating pinwheel. Entrainment mapping is like putting your finger in the pinwheel and spinning it slightly faster and then removing it. Pacing from sites away from the reentrant circuit will yield flutter waves that are different than during tachycardia (Fig. 12.5). In addition, because of the time required for depolarization to travel to and from the reentrant circuit, the return cycle length after the final paced beat will be longer. The closer one moves the pacing

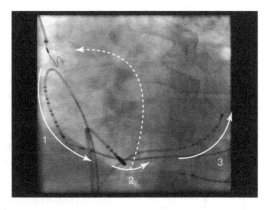

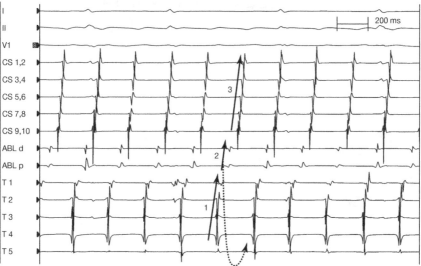

Figure 12.4 Electrograms from a patient with typical atrial flutter. Atrial depolarization travels from superior to inferior down the lateral wall of the right atrium (1) and can be seen in the decapolar catheter placed in the right atrium (T1–T5). Temporally the next portion of atrial activation is seen in the ablation/mapping (ABL) catheter in the cavotricuspid isthmus (2). Atrial depolarization then splits, activating the coronary sinus (CS) electrodes (3) and the septal wall of the right atrium (dashed arrow in the fluoroscopic image, not shown in the EGM).

site to the reentrant circuit the less different the flutter waves will look, and the return cycle length of the last paced beat will become shorter. When pacing is performed within the reentrant circuit, the flutter waves will look the same as during tachycardia (since the atria are being activated in the same fashion), but the flutter waves will be separated by the paced interval. In addition, when pacing from the reentrant circuit, the return cycle of the last paced beat will match the tachycardia cycle length (since they took the same path). Using these techniques, the location of a reentrant circuit can be identified. Entrainment mapping is used to determine whether the cavotricuspid isthmus is critical to the tachycardia circuit by pacing from the cavotricuspid isthmus (Fig. 12.6).

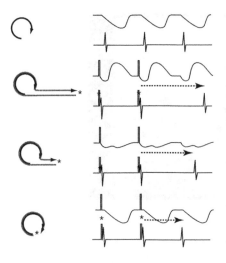

Figure 12.5 Theoretical effects of pacing during tachycardia (entrainment) in atrial flutter. Pacing is performed at a rate slightly faster than the tachycardia cycle length. As the distance between the pacing site and the reentrant circuit is decreased the paced flutter waves will look more like the tachycardia flutter waves, and the return cycle length after the last paced beat will become shorter. When pacing is performed from within the reentrant circuit the paced beats will have the same morphology as the tachycardia beats, and the return cycle length will match the tachycardia cycle length.

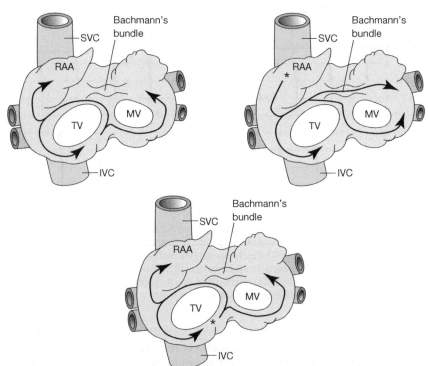

Figure 12.6 Schematic showing atrial flutter (top left) and the effects of pacing from different atrial sites (*). When pacing from outside the circuit (top right), the flutter waves due to paced beats will exhibit a different morphology from the atrial flutter. However, pacing from the cavotricuspid isthmus (bottom) will produce flutter waves that match the tachycardia. IVC, inferior vena cava; MV, mitral valve; RAA, right atrial appendage; SVC, superior vena cava; TV, tricuspid valve. (Adapted with permission from Kusumoto FM. *Cardiovascular Pathophysiology*. Raleigh, NC: Hayes Barton Press, 1999.)

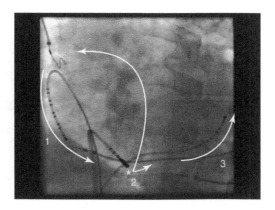

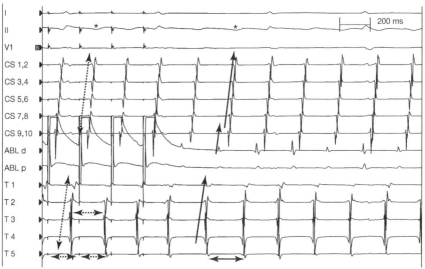

Figure 12.7 The same patient as Fig. 12.4. Pacing from the cavotricuspid isthmus at a rate slightly faster than the tachycardia rate (double-headed arrows) produces flutter waves (*) and intracardiac electrograms (single-headed arrows) that are the same as those observed in tachycardia. Dashed arrows, pacing; solid arrows, tachycardia.

In the same patient as Fig. 12.4, the effects of pacing from the cavotricuspid isthmus are shown in Fig. 12.7. Pacing from the cavotricuspid isthmus produces flutter waves that are exactly the same as the flutter waves in tachycardia. As a surrogate, since the subtleties of flutter waves can be difficult to assess, the intracardiac electrograms can be used. In this patient, pacing at a rate (double-headed dashed arrows) slightly faster than the tachycardia rate leads to more rapid atrial activation. Since the pacing is performed at the critical isthmus used in the tachycardia circuit the flutter waves (*) and the atrial electrograms are similar during pacing (dashed single arrows) and tachycardia (solid single arrows).

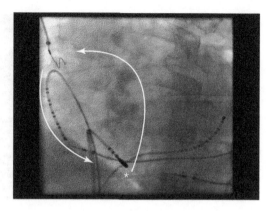

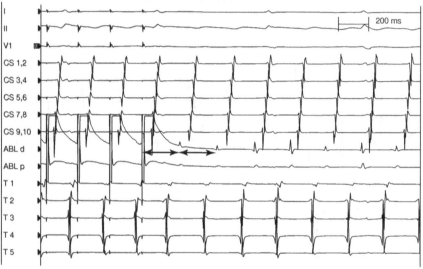

Figure 12.8 On cessation of pacing the return cycle length from the last paced beat to the electrogram recorded from that site (post-pacing interval) matches the tachycardia cycle length (since they took the same path). This finding suggests that the pacing site is part of the reentrant circuit.

In addition to the atrial activation pattern, the return cycle length after the last paced beat can be evaluated. As discussed previously, the farther pacing is performed from the critical isthmus used for tachycardia, the longer the return cycle length will be. However, when pacing is performed from within the circuit, the return cycle length from the pacing stimulus to the electrogram from the pacing site (the post-pacing interval or PPI) will be equal to the tachycardia cycle length. In Fig. 12.8, the return cycle length is equal to the tachycardia cycle length at the cavotricuspid isthmus.

Most commonly, atrial flutter travels through the cavotricuspid isthmus in a lateral-to-medial direction. In some cases, however, atrial depolarization through the isthmus occurs in the medial-to-lateral direction. Figure 12.9

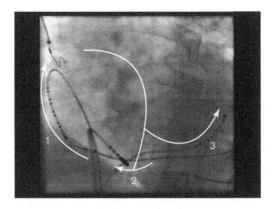

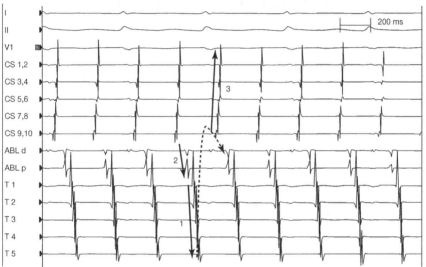

Figure 12.9 Electrograms from an atrial flutter traveling in the opposite direction, from the patient illustrated in Figs. 12.4, 12.7, and 12.8. Since the flutter circuit is the same distance (just reversed direction), the cycle lengths of the two tachycardias are the same. In this case activation of the lateral wall of the right atrium proceeds from inferior to superior. This type of flutter is also called *clockwise atrial flutter*, in reference to the reversed direction.

shows this "unusual" form of typical atrial flutter, from the same patient illustrated in Figs. 12.4, 12.7, and 12.8. Notice that the atrial depolarization pattern is completely reversed in the lateral wall but the tachycardia cycle length is the same as in Fig. 12.4. This type of atrial flutter is called the *unusual form* of typical atrial flutter, or *clockwise atrial flutter*. A 12-lead ECG during tachycardia is shown in Fig. 12.10. Reversed atrial activation leads to less prominent flutter waves in the inferior leads.

In all forms of cavotricuspid isthmus-dependent atrial flutter, ablation is performed by placing a series of lesions that span this critical isthmus. Ablation

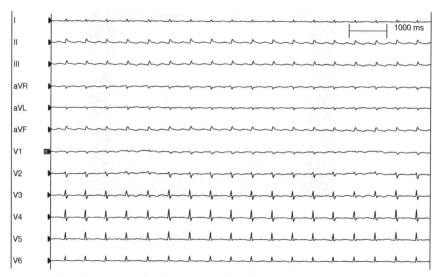

Figure 12.10 ECG during clockwise atrial flutter. The typical negative flutter waves in the inferior leads are no longer observed.

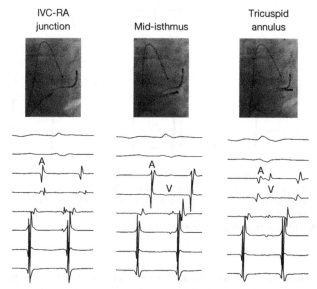

Figure 12.11 During ablation for atrial flutter, a series of lesions are placed from the tricuspid valve to the inferior vena cava in an attempt to create a line of block that spans the cavotricuspid isthmus.

lesions are placed from the tricuspid valve to the inferior vena cava (Fig. 12.11). The location of the ablation catheter can be estimated by evaluating the relative electrogram sizes of the ventricular and atrial signals. It is important to keep several anatomic considerations in mind when performing ablation in this

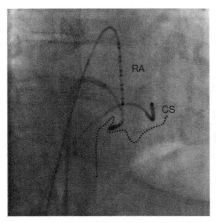
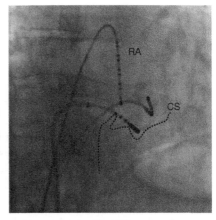

Eustachian Ridge   "Pouch"

Figure 12.12 In many patients with atrial flutter, creation of a line of block requires "curling under" the eustachian ridge that separates the inferior vena cava from the inferior right atrium and ablating within "pouches" or deep sulci within the isthmus itself.

region. First, the eustachian ridge is a "floppy" wall that is located at the posterior border of the isthmus separating the inferior vena cava and the inferior right atrium. As ablation is performed, the presence of this structure will often not be appreciated by simply "dragging" the catheter back. Unless the catheter is curled back, the most posterior portion of the isthmus will not be ablated. In addition, the isthmus can often have pouches and crevices that require ablation. Examples of a deep pouch and ablating under the eustachian ridge are shown in Fig. 12.12.

When performing ablation for atrial flutter it is important to remember that AV block can occur in approximately 1% of cases, and it is important for the clinician to monitor the frequency of the QRS complexes as ablation is performed. It is always reassuring to see variable conduction intervals 2 : 1 interspersed with 3 : 1 activation, because this implies that some AV conduction is present. The development of regular relatively slow QRS rates should always arouse suspicion for accompanying AV node injury. Ablation can be performed in any region of the cavotricuspid isthmus. It may be that ablation at regions "away" from the septum may be associated with a reduced risk of AV block.

Atrial flutter will often terminate as the ablation is performed (Fig. 12.13). However, it is important to remember that the goal for ablation is to produce a "line of block" that spans a region from the tricuspid valve to the inferior vena cava. The end point for ablation of atrial flutter is not to identify a single focus but rather to transect the critical isthmus required for sustaining reentry. Pacing maneuvers and evaluation of the temporal and spatial patterns of atrial activation are used to determine whether block in the cavotricuspid isthmus has been achieved (Fig. 12.14). In the second row, pacing from the coronary

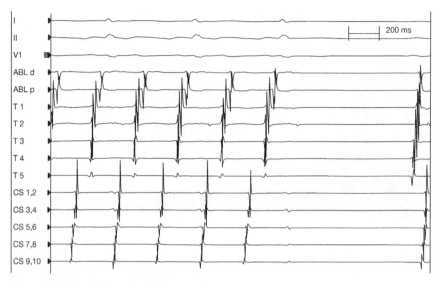

Figure 12.13 Termination of atrial flutter as ablation is being performed and a lesion is placed at the inferior vena cava–right atrial junction under the eustachian ridge. Notice the large atrial component and absent ventricular electrogram on the ablation catheter (ABL).

sinus is performed. Notice that although depolarization is "slow" through the isthmus, atrial depolarization still travels through the region to excite the lateral wall of the right atrium. In this case, although atrial flutter has been abolished the substrate for reentry still exists. Further ablation, perhaps under the eustachian ridge or in a deep pouch, is required. The third row shows the same patient after cavotricuspid isthmus block has been achieved. Notice that the activation pattern in the lateral wall of the right atrium has been completely reversed. As a consequence the interval between the electrograms recorded at the coronary sinus and a catheter located just lateral to the line of block has increased substantially. The fourth row shows that block is also present in the opposite direction. Pacing from lateral to the ablation line is performed, and atrial depolarization must travel superiorly up the lateral wall of the right atrium and down the septal wall to reach the coronary sinus.

Figure 12.14 (*opposite*) Evaluation of conduction through the cavotricuspid isthmus during tachycardia (top row) and after ablation (second through fourth rows). The ablation catheter has been moved to a position just lateral to the site of ablation (dots). *Second row:* After termination of atrial flutter, pacing (*) from the coronary sinus shows that conduction is still present in the cavotricuspid isthmus. Although the conduction interval across the isthmus is prolonged, the lateral wall of the right atrium is still activated via the cavotricuspid isthmus. *Third row:* After additional ablation, true cavotricuspid isthmus block is now present. Pacing from the coronary sinus produces superior-to-inferior depolarization of the lateral right atrial wall, with latest depolarization of the ablation catheter. *Fourth row:* Pacing from just lateral to the right atrium is associated with inferior to superior activation of the right atrium before activation of the coronary sinus because of the presence of cavotricuspid isthmus block. CS, coronary sinus; LLRA, low lateral right atrium.

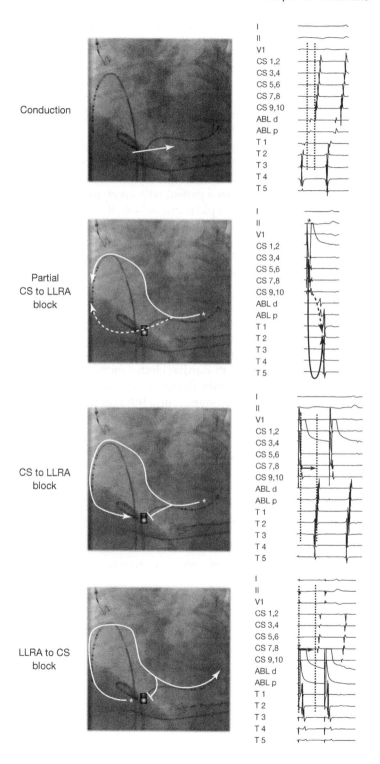

Conduction

Partial
CS to LLRA
block

CS to LLRA
block

LLRA to CS
block

Cavotricupid isthmus-independent atrial flutter

Atrial flutters can involve critical regions that are away from the cavotricuspid isthmus. It is important to be aware that non-isthmus-dependent atrial flutters also commonly use barriers/scar to form a critical isthmus. The clinician must always keep in mind possible structures that may be involved in the flutter circuit: mitral valve, prior surgery/atriotomy (such as atrial septal defect repair), or prior ablations. Evaluation of the flutter waves on the ECG can be very helpful for evaluating the general pattern of depolarization. Unfortunately, atrial flutters that do not involve the cavotricuspid isthmus often have very attenuated flutter waves, particularly if they are within the left atrium. Figure 12.15 shows the ECG from a patient with an atypical atrial flutter that is not dependent on the cavotricuspid isthmus. Note that the flutter waves are negative in the inferior leads, illustrating that the surface ECG is rather limited for identifying the location of the reentrant circuit.

When confronted with a patient with a cavotricuspid isthmus-independent flutter the clinician must use entrainment mapping techniques to identify the components of the reentrant circuit. The intracardiac electrograms from the patient from Fig. 12.15 are shown in Fig. 12.16. Electrograms can be seen spanning the entire cycle length, suggesting that the tachycardia is a macro-reentrant atrial flutter.

Identification of the important components of the reentrant circuit requires a methodical evaluation of the intracardiac electrograms. First, determination of the "diastolic" period between the flutter waves can provide an initial clue for the location of the "critical isthmus," since this region will often be "ECG

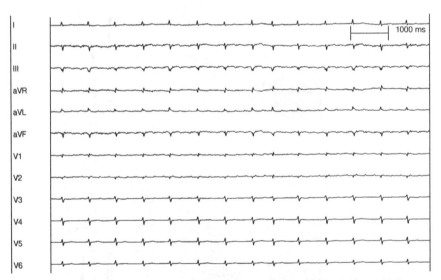

Figure 12.15 ECG from a patient with cavotricuspid isthmus-independent atrial flutter. Notice that the flutter waves are negative in the inferior leads.

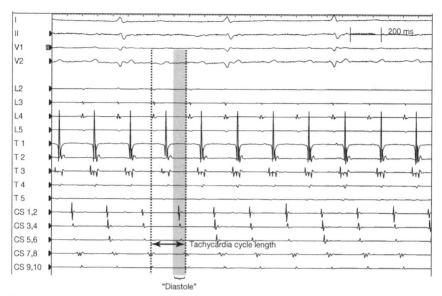

Figure 12.16 Intracardiac electrograms from the patient in Fig. 12.15. Decapolar catheters are located in the coronary sinus (CS), the lateral wall of the right atrium (T1–T5), and the posterior left atrium near the left upper pulmonary vein (L1–L5).

silent." Similar to mapping focal atrial tachycardias, it is worthwhile to examine all 12 ECG leads to find the lead with the most prominent P wave. In this case, lead V_2 demonstrated the largest P waves, and this lead is displayed and "gained up," allowing identification of the diastolic period; inspection of the electrograms shows that coronary sinus activation occurs during this time, suggesting that this may be an important region involved in the reentrant circuit. Review Fig. 12.4, and notice that the electrograms from the cavotricuspid isthmus also correlate with the "isoelectric" or "diastolic" period between the negative flutter waves. Depolarization of the critical isthmus of a reentrant circuit is often isoelectric on the surface ECG, since a small portion of the atria is being activated during this period. Although electrogram timing in relation to the flutter waves is useful, careful entrainment techniques are necessary for confirmation of a critical isthmus. In Fig. 12.17, the effects of pacing from the lateral right atrial wall, distal coronary sinus, and posterior left atrium near the left upper pulmonary vein are shown. Since the return cycle is longest from the lateral wall of the right atrium, and shorter from both left atrial sites, the tachycardia circuit is located within the left atrium. Since the return cycle length of the coronary sinus electrogram almost matches the tachycardia cycle length, the anterior left atrium near the mitral valve is probably an important component of the tachycardia circuit. Figure 12.18 diagrammatically shows the effects of changes in pacing site on the return cycle length of the last paced beat during entrainment mapping.

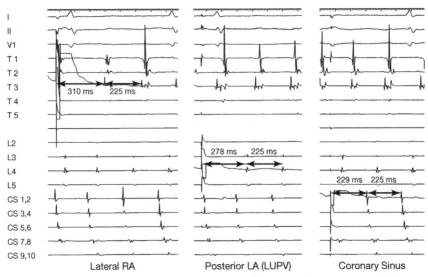

Figure 12.17 Entrainment techniques to identify the general location of a reentrant circuit. Pacing from the right atrium (RA) results in the longest post-pacing interval, suggesting that the reentrant circuit is confined to the left atrium (LA). The shortest post-pacing interval is observed with coronary sinus pacing, which provides important evidence that this region should be carefully evaluated. LUPV, left upper pulmonary vein.

A mapping catheter is now moved to the endocardial surface of the left atrium in this region and pacing is repeated (Figs. 12.19, 12.20). An electrogram that is in the diastolic period is recorded from the distal tip of a decapolar catheter placed on the endocardial surface of the left atrium. Pacing from this site results in a post-pacing interval that matches the tachycardia. The surface P wave (best seen in V₂) and the atrial endocardial activation pattern are the same for both pacing and tachycardia. Finally, the interval from stimulus to P wave matches that from endocardial electrogram to P wave (62 ms).

Once the critical isthmus for the reentrant circuit is identified, an ablation strategy can be planned. Angiography shows the relationship between the left-sided pulmonary veins and the mitral annulus (approximated by the position of the coronary sinus catheter) (Fig. 12.21). Ablation is performed by placing a series of ablation lesions from the mitral annulus to the base of the left inferior pulmonary vein. As the ablation line is completed, termination of the atrial flutter occurs (Fig. 12.22). As in the case for cavotricuspid isthmus-dependent flutter, pacing must be performed on either side of the ablation line to confirm block (Fig. 12.23).

Three-dimensional mapping technology facilitates ablation of atrial flutter by allowing the clinician to identify and tag specific anatomic sites and reliably return to those sites later in the case. However, it is important that the clinician uses information from three-dimensional mapping as a supplement to information obtained from intracardiac electrograms. A strategy for mapping and

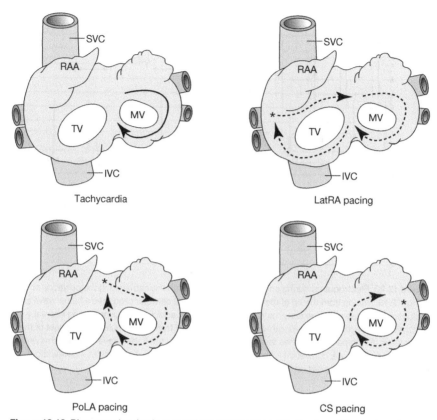

Tachycardia

LatRA pacing

PoLA pacing

CS pacing

Figure 12.18 Diagrams showing how entrainment mapping and evaluation of the post-pacing interval helps identify the location of the tachycardia circuit. The farther away a pacing site (*) is from the reentrant circuit, the longer the post-pacing interval will be. LatRA, lateral right atrium; PoLA, posterior left atrium; CS, coronary sinus. Other abbreviations as in Fig. 12.6. (Adapted from Kusumoto FM. *Cardiovascular Pathophysiology*. Raleigh, NC: Hayes Barton Press, 1999).

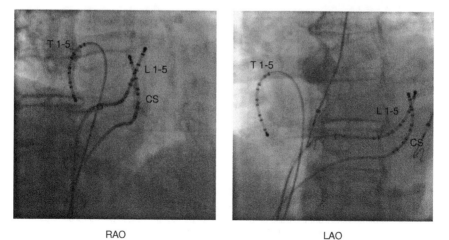

RAO

LAO

Figure 12.19 The decapolar catheter originally placed in the posterior left atrium has now been moved to the endocardial surface of the left atrium overlying the coronary sinus (L1–5).

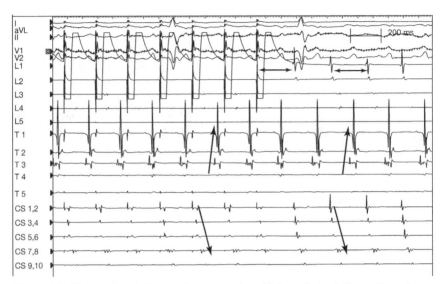

Figure 12.20 Electrograms during entrainment mapping with the catheters in the positions shown in Fig. 12.18. Pacing from the tip of the endocardial left atrial catheter produces a flutter wave and endocardial activation that exactly matches tachycardia. In addition, the post-pacing interval matches the tachycardia cycle length, and third, the interval from the stimulus to the onset of the flutter wave during pacing matches the interval to the onset of the flutter wave during tachycardia. All of these findings are consistent with the critical isthmus for a reentrant circuit. Abbreviations correspond to catheter positions shown in Fig. 12.19.

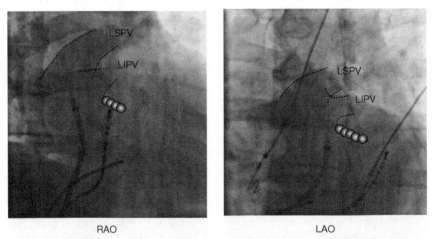

Figure 12.21 Angiograms of the left atrium and left pulmonary veins in the right anterior oblique (RAO) and left anterior oblique (LAO) projections. Based on entrainment mapping it was elected to place an ablation line from the base of the left inferior pulmonary vein to the mitral annulus. LSPV, left superior pulmonary vein; LIPV, left inferior pulmonary vein.

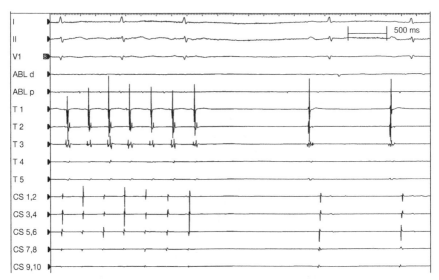

Figure 12.22 As ablation from the mitral valve to the left inferior pulmonary vein is performed, termination of the atrial flutter is observed.

ablating patients with atrial flutter is summarized in Figs. 12.24 and 12.25. In general it is very helpful to start "global" (surface ECG evaluation), gradually move "regionally" (left or right atrium, anterior or posterior portions of the heart), and ultimately end up "in the neighborhood" (identification of a critical isthmus facilitated by three-dimensional mapping). The one exception is to always look first for "common things," and to determine whether a flutter is dependent on the cavotricuspid isthmus by using entrainment mapping.

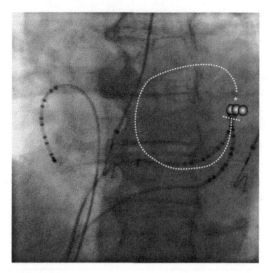

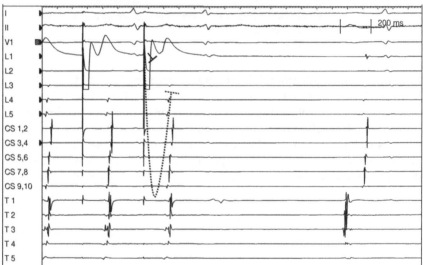

Figure 12.23 Pacing from a site superior to the ablation line confirms the presence of conduction block with delayed activation of the distal coronary sinus and a proximal-to-distal conduction pattern in the coronary sinus (dotted line in the fluoroscopic images and the electrograms).

What structural issues may be clinically relevant?
• Prior cardiac surgery – Location of incisions and artificial
  material
• Congenital heart disease
• Prior ablations

Flutter wave morphology
• Identify the general direction of depolarization
• Guess the origin of depolarization

Is the flutter dependent on the cavotricuspid isthmus?
• Perform entrainment mapping at the cavotricuspid isthmus

Left or right atrium?
• Entrainment mapping from left and right atrial sites and identify
  the atrium associated with the shortest post pacing intervals

Identification of the critical isthmus
• Entrainment mapping: start regionally and gradually decrease
  the area of interest.
• Use 3-dimensional mapping to facilitate location of the isthmus
• Plan an effective ablation strategy

Figure 12.24 Flowchart for evaluation of atrial flutter in the electrophysiology laboratory.

Pacing from sites far away from the reentrant circuit:
1. Will produce flutter waves and endocardial activation patterns that are
   different than tachycardia
2. Long post pacing intervals

Pacing from closer sites:
1. Will produce flutter waves and endocardial activation patterns that are more
   similar to tachycardia
2. Shorten the postpacing intervals

Pacing from within the critical isthmus:
1. Will result in flutter waves and endocardial activation that match tachycardia
2. Postpacing interval will match the tachycardia cycle length
3. The stimulus to P wave interval will match the electrogram to P wave interval
4. Endocardial potential will be present in the "diastolic" period

Figure 12.25 Summary of entrainment mapping techniques.

CHAPTER 13

Atrial fibrillation

Atrial fibrillation is the most commonly observed arrhythmia in clinical medicine. In the United States it is estimated that over 5 million people have atrial fibrillation, and because of the aging of our population the prevalence of this arrhythmia will increase significantly over the next decade. Despite its prevalence, at least in part because of complexity, very few groups and clinicians studied possible therapeutic options for atrial fibrillation. However, in the 1980s the group at Washington University devised a surgical procedure called the "Maze" that was successful for the treatment of atrial fibrillation. In a landmark paper in the mid-1990s, Haissaguerre and colleagues reported on the importance of pulmonary vein triggers for the initiation of atrial fibrillation. Since then there has been an explosion of studies evaluating nonpharmacologic treatment of atrial fibrillation; in 2008 alone there were more than 700 studies on atrial fibrillation ablation. Ablation for atrial fibrillation is now the most commonly performed procedure in our laboratory.

Mechanism

Despite its prevalence and importance, even after more than 100 years of research by numerous investigators, the mechanisms for atrial fibrillation remain incompletely understood. It is likely that there are multiple causes, including multiple changing wavelets, or small reentrant circuits, or rapidly firing foci associated with fibrillatory conduction. Fibrillatory conduction appears to develop because of regions of block and refractoriness within the atria. To make matters even more complex, each of these cellular mechanisms can involve different tissue types including the pulmonary vein, posterior left atrium, and other sites. Finally, any mechanism for atrial fibrillation can be modulated by the sympathetic and parasympathetic system, and by changes in atrial tissue architecture over time.

Electrocardiogram

The ECG in atrial fibrillation shows irregular waves due to chaotic activation of the atria (Fig. 13.1). Although investigators have studied the characteristics

---

Understanding Intracardiac EGMs and ECGs. By Fred Kusumoto. Published 2010 by Blackwell Publishing. ISBN: 978-1-4051-8410-6

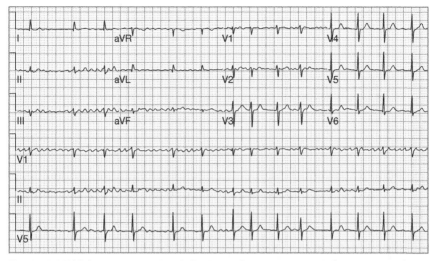

Figure 13.1 ECG from a patient with atrial fibrillation. Chaotic atrial activity (fibrillatory waves) can be observed in all of the ECG leads.

of fibrillatory waves, in general the ECG has provided little information on the pathophysiology of the disease.

Electrophysiology

Interest in the electrophysiology of atrial fibrillation dramatically increased in the 1990s when it was recognized that rapid atrial tachycardias or single premature atrial contractions from the pulmonary vein could initiate atrial fibrillation. An example of this phenomenon is shown in Figs. 13.2 and 13.3. In this case a multipolar basket catheter similar to the one shown in Fig. 11.14 (Chapter 11) has been placed in the left superior pulmonary vein. Electrograms

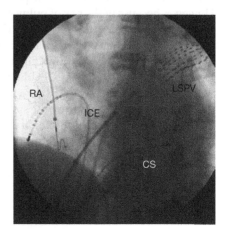

Figure 13.2 A basket catheter has been placed in the left superior pulmonary vein (LSPV). Decapolar catheters are placed in the coronary sinus (CS) and the lateral wall of the right atrium (RA). An intracardiac echocardiography (ICE) catheter marks the interatrial septum.

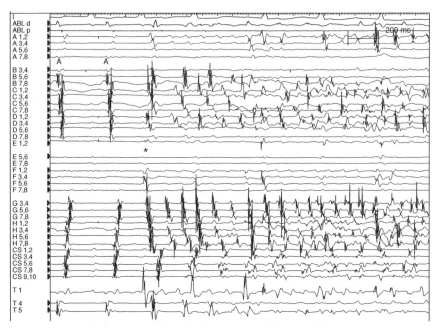

Figure 13.3 Electrograms from the patient shown in Fig. 13.2. Letters A–H identify the splines of the basket catheter, with the more proximal electrode pairs numbered 5,6 and 7,8. Rapid focal activation from electrodes 3,4 in the B spline, and additional early activation noted at electrodes 3,4 on the F spline (*), suddenly initiates irregular activation within the pulmonary vein and the development of atrial fibrillation. A, atrial activation due to sinus rhythm.

reveal an atrial tachycardia from the pulmonary vein, which deteriorates into atrial fibrillation. There are a number of techniques that have been described for ablation of atrial fibrillation, but most center on ablation of the pulmonary vein region.

Initially, trigger sites within the pulmonary vein were targeted for ablation. However, because of the risk of pulmonary vein stenosis and recurrent arrhythmias from other sites, the strategy shifted to making a circumferential lesion around the pulmonary veins in an attempt to isolate rapid activity within the veins from the rest of the atrium (Fig. 13.4) by a series of point-by-point lesions. Figure 13.5 shows an isolated pulmonary vein, with rapid depolarizations within the pulmonary vein that are not conducted to the atria. The patient's atria are activated normally by the sinus node.

Although isolating the pulmonary veins is effective in some patients, it is now appreciated that sites within the left atrium may be important for the development or maintenance of atrial fibrillation in a large number of patients. In addition, regions of high-frequency atrial activity – often referred to as *complex fractionated atrial electrograms* or CFAEs – have also been targets for ablation, particularly in those patients with persistent atrial fibrillation. Although definitions vary, CFAEs are characterized by short cycle lengths (< 120 ms)

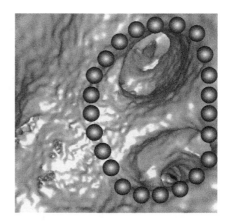

Figure 13.4 Endoscopic view of the right pulmonary veins. Ablation is performed by moving an ablation catheter in a point-by-point manner to isolate the pulmonary veins.

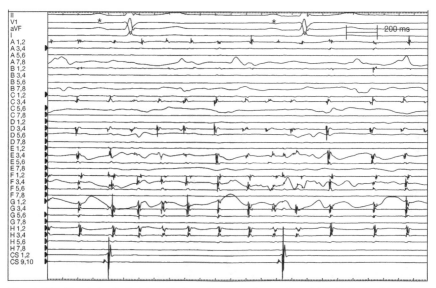

Figure 13.5 A basket catheter placed in the pulmonary vein reveals atrial fibrillation/rapid atrial activity. However, depolarization is blocked at the pulmonary vein–left atrial junction and the atria are activated normally by the sinus node (*).

and low-voltage signals with varying amplitudes (0.06–0.25 mV). In Fig. 13.6, CFAEs from the roof of the left atrium are identified. Notice that rapid depolarization at the roof of the left atrium is associated with regular activation of the coronary sinus region, again emphasizing the importance of the careful mapping required in any patient with any atrial tachycardia. Almost any region of the atria can have CFAEs, but they appear to be clustered in particular sites such as the interatrial septum, posterior left atrium, left atrial roof, or the floor of the left atrium for individual patients.

For ablation of the pulmonary veins, traditionally point ablations around the pulmonary veins are performed, guided by fluoroscopy or an advanced

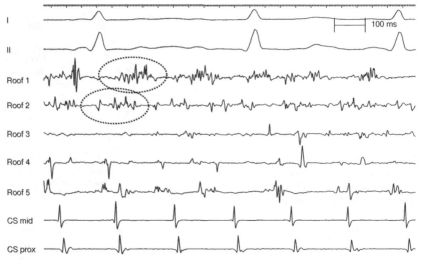

Figure 13.6 Complex fractionated atrial electrograms (CFAEs) recorded from the roof of the left atrium (ellipses) in a patient with persistent atrial fibrillation. CFAEs are characterized by rapid fractionated electrograms with varying amplitude.

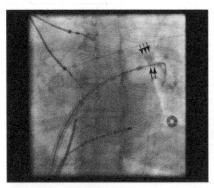

Figure 13.7 Balloon designed to deliver cryoablation at the pulmonary vein os. The wire is located in a lower branch of the left superior pulmonary vein. The balloon is occluding the vein, as evidenced by contrast "hanging up" within the vein (arrows).

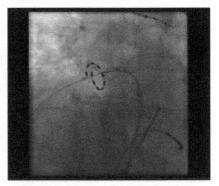

Figure 13.8 A circular catheter designed to deliver radiofrequency energy at all of the electrodes has been placed in the right superior vein. A guidewire has been placed through the catheter onto the vein to help stabilize the catheter position.

mapping system. However, even with the newest technology, ablation can be time-intensive and difficult. Several manufacturers have developed catheters for ablating larger regions around the pulmonary veins, including balloons or circular ablation catheters. A balloon-based system is shown in Fig. 13.7. In this case cryoenergy delivered on the surface of the balloon is used to isolate the pulmonary veins. Figure 13.8 shows a multielectrode circular ablation catheter that is designed to deliver radiofrequency energy at all of the electrodes placed in the right superior pulmonary vein. Figure 13.9 shows the electrograms

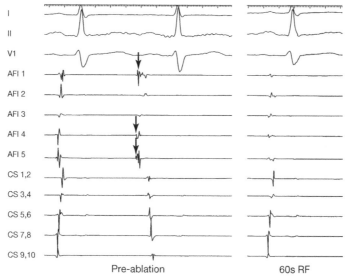

Figure 13.9 Electrograms from the catheter position in Fig. 13.8. *Left:* At baseline, pulmonary vein potentials can be seen (arrows), which also initiate a premature atrial complex. *Right:* After radiofrequency (RF) ablation, pulmonary vein potentials are eliminated. Only signals from adjacent atrial tissue are recorded.

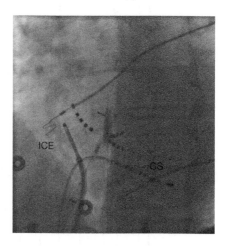

Figure 13.10 A specially designed "winged" catheter is placed on the left atrial side of the interatrial septum.

before and after application of radiofrequency energy. Notice that pulmonary vein potentials have been eliminated with a single ablation.

Specialized catheters are being developed to ablate several sites within the left atrium at once. Since CFAEs are often identified on the interatrial septum, one design uses a catheter with retractable "winged electrodes" that can be deployed against the left atrial side of the interatrial septum to perform ablation (Fig. 13.10). Electrograms before and after ablation with this catheter design are shown in Fig. 13.11. The complex fractionated atrial activity that is observed before treatment is significantly attenuated with ablation.

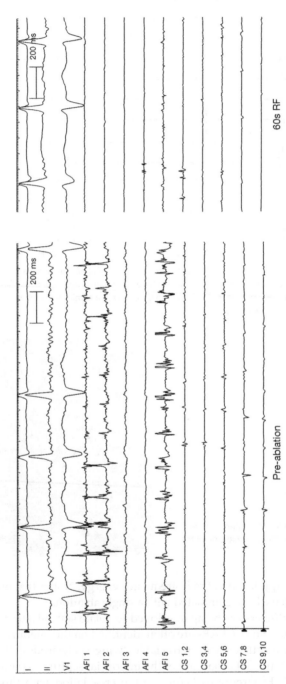

Figure 13.11 Intracardiac electrograms obtained from the catheter position in Fig. 13.10. Prior to ablation, salvos of complex fractionated atrial electrograms are observed. After radiofrequency (RF) ablation, the signals are attenuated and there is no evidence of rapid atrial activity.

CHAPTER 14

Ventricular tachycardia

Electrophysiology testing and ablation of ventricular arrhythmias can be extremely challenging. However, tremendous progress over the past 5–10 years, built on seminal work from surgical studies in the 1970s, has increased the applicability of electrophysiology and, in particular, ablation as an adjunctive therapy for the treatment of ventricular arrhythmias. In addition, greater use of implantable cardioverter defibrillators and recognition of the deleterious effects of inappropriate shocks has further increased the use of ablation in patients with, or even simply at risk for, ventricular arrhythmias.

Mechanism

It is important to determine the mechanism of the ventricular arrhythmia. It is obvious that the ablation strategy for arrhythmia due to a "point source" will be different from that used for a reentrant circuit. Ventricular tachycardia in the setting of no structural heart disease is almost always due to abnormal automaticity or triggered activity. In contrast, in patients with structural heart disease reentry is the most common mechanism for ventricular tachycardia, due to the presence of "patchy scars" that increase the likelihood of "protected channels" forming the substrate for reentry.

Electrophysiology testing can provide clues to the mechanism for tachycardia. Induction of ventricular tachycardia with premature ventricular extrastimuli suggests an underlying reentrant mechanism, although triggered activity can also be initiated this way. Figure 14.1 shows a typical example of stable ventricular tachycardia initiated with two ventricular extrastimuli. In contrast, initiation of ventricular tachycardia due to automaticity is often rate-related and is usually performed by ventricular pacing or atrial pacing at a constant rate. In addition, isoproterenol is often required to initiate the tachycardia. Figure 14.2 shows initiation of ventricular tachycardia with constant ventricular pacing at a cycle length of 350 ms. Figure 6.9 (Chapter 6) shows an example of ventricular tachycardia initiated by atrial pacing. In both examples notice that ventricular tachycardia is confirmed because of the presence of atrioventricular dissociation.

In patients with structural heart disease due to prior myocardial infarction, one of the traditional uses for electrophysiologic testing was to evaluate risk of

Understanding Intracardiac EGMs and ECGs. By Fred Kusumoto. Published 2010 by Blackwell Publishing. ISBN: 978-1-4051-8410-6

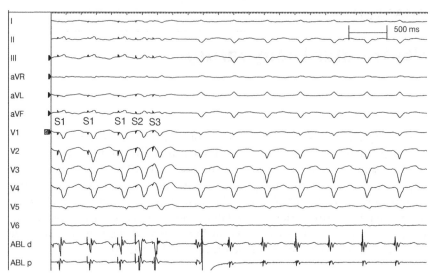

Figure 14.1 Initiation of ventricular tachycardia with two premature ventricular extrastimuli (S_2 and S_3).

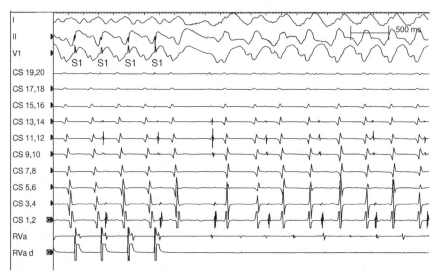

Figure 14.2 Initiation of ventricular tachycardia with ventricular pacing at a cycle length of 350 ms (S_1). Ventricular tachycardia is confirmed by the presence of more QRS complexes than atrial electrograms.

ventricular arrhythmias for a specific patient. With the advent of the widespread use of implantable cardioverter defibrillators, use of electrophysiologic testing for this indication has declined, but it is important to remember that electrophysiologic testing remains an important test with excellent negative predictive value in selected patients. This means that if a patient is non-inducible for sustained ventricular arrhythmias despite multiple ventricular extrastimuli (negative study), the likelihood of future sudden cardiac death is very low. The most common cause of ventricular arrhythmias in patients with prior myocardial infarction is reentrant ventricular tachycardia, which can usually be reliably reproduced with ventricular extrastimuli. Although ventricular extrastimulation protocols vary, a common technique is summarized in Fig. 14.3. The ventricular effective refractory period is determined with a single ventricular extrastimulus. Double extrastimuli are now delivered,

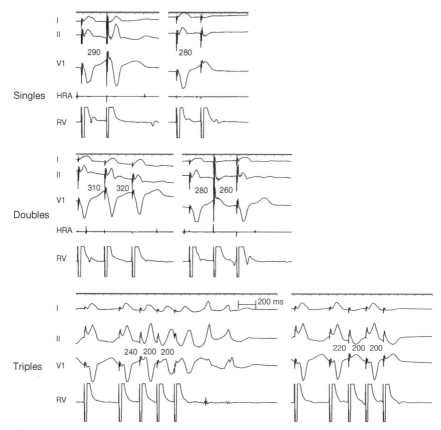

Figure 14.3 Ventricular extrastimulation protocol for initiating reentrant ventricular arrhythmias and assessing risk for sudden cardiac death. First, single extrastimuli are delivered at incrementally shorter intervals until the ventricular effective refractory period (VERP) is reached (top row). Double extrastimuli (middle row) are delivered, initially using coupling intervals 30–40 ms greater than VERP. The extrastimuli are coupled shorter and shorter (usually S_3 before S_2) until the second extrastimulus does not capture. Triple extrastimuli are then delivered (bottom row). With triple extrastimuli, nonsustained salvos of polymorphic ventricular tachycardia will often be observed. The protocol is finished when the coupling interval reach 200 ms or ventricular capture is lost on the first and third extrastimuli.

usually starting with coupling intervals 30–40 ms greater than the ventricular effective refractory period (doubles). Extrastimuli are gradually delivered earlier and earlier in increments of 10 ms (to a minimal interval of 200 ms in our laboratory). Once the second extrastimulus reaches ventricular effective refractory period, three extrastimuli are delivered. The three extrastimuli are usually initially programmed to coupling intervals 30–40 ms above the ventricular effective refractory period and progressively the third, second, and first extrastimuli are coupled earlier and earlier. With triple extrastimuli it is frequent to produce nonsustained salvos of polymorphic ventricular tachycardia (Fig. 14.3). The extrastimulation protocol is finished when the coupling intervals reach 200 ms or the patient develops refractoriness in the first and third extrastimuli (S_2 and S_4 block). Multiple studies have shown that inability to induce sustained ventricular arrhythmias (> 30 ms) despite this protocol using two different drive cycles and pacing from two different sites is associated with a very low risk for sudden cardiac death.

Once ventricular tachycardia is initiated it is important to first evaluate the clinical status of the patient. In Fig. 14.4, triple ventricular extrastimuli lead to initiation of rapid polymorphic ventricular tachycardia/ventricular fibrillation. It is very unlikely that this tachycardia will be hemodynamically tolerated, and preparations for defibrillation should begin immediately. Invasive hemodynamic monitoring of central arterial pressure can be very helpful, particularly in those patients with structural heart disease. Figure 14.5 shows an example of a patient with induction of ventricular tachycardia. Although there is some beat-to-beat alteration in systemic blood pressure, overall the tracings

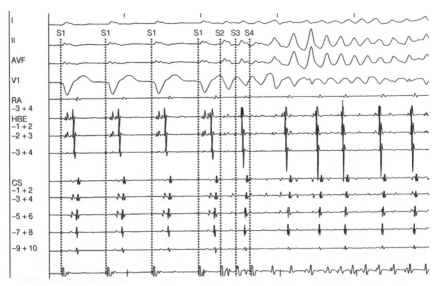

Figure 14.4 Initiation of polymorphic ventricular tachycardia/ventricular fibrillation with triple extrastimuli (S_2, S_3, and S_4).

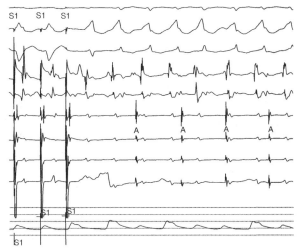

Figure 14.5 Initiation of ventricular tachycardia (atrioventricular dissociation is present). Even in ventricular tachycardia systolic blood pressure ranges from 80 to 110 mmHg. A, atrial electrogram.

confirm relative hemodynamic stability. In addition, in our laboratory, if the patient is receiving conscious sedation a staff member is constantly monitoring the mental status of the patient and determining whether symptoms such as chest pain are present.

In patients with structural heart disease it is often useful to evaluate the response of the ventricular tachycardia to pacing. Pacing can be associated with several responses: continuation of the tachycardia, acceleration of the tachycardia, or termination of the tachycardia. Figure 14.6 shows an example of pace-termination of ventricular tachycardia. When performing ventricular pacing it is obviously important to confirm capture both by evaluating the local ventricular electrogram and by noting a change in the QRS complex. Rapid ventricular pacing can also accelerate the ventricular tachycardia (Fig. 14.7), and in some cases induce ventricular fibrillation (Fig. 14.8). Figure 14.9 shows a schematic of potential mechanisms for some of the possible outcomes associated with ventricular pacing during ventricular tachycardia. Ventricular tachycardia in patients with structural heart disease is usually due to development of a reentrant circuit that uses channels formed by patchy scars. If ventricular depolarization can enter both the exit and entrance of the reentrant circuit, when pacing is stopped the tachycardia terminates. If ventricular depolarization does not interact with the reentrant circuit, or enters only the exit site, when pacing is stopped the last depolarization wave can then continue the tachycardia if it does not encounter refractory tissue. Acceleration of ventricular tachycardia can occur if the ventricular pacing results in the development of another reentrant circuit.

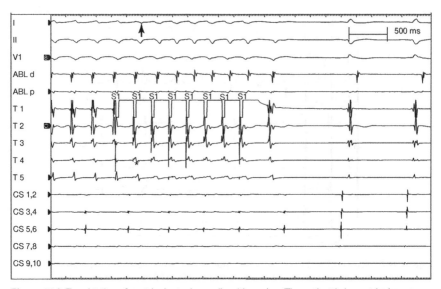

Figure 14.6 Termination of ventricular tachycardia with pacing. The patient is in ventricular tachycardia at a cycle length of 280 ms. Ventricular pacing is performed at 230 ms (S_1). The second and subsequent S_1 extrastmuli result in ventricular capture (* on the local electrogram, arrow marking the change in the QRS complex). On cessation of pacing, ventricular tachycardia is no longer present.

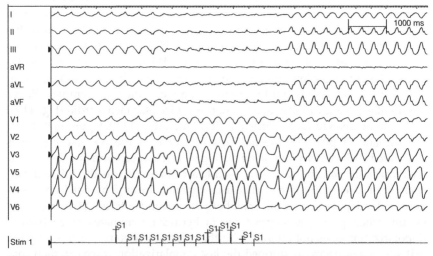

Figure 14.7 Ventricular pacing accelerates ventricular tachycardia. During ventricular tachycardia, burst pacing is associated with effective ventricular capture (note the change in the QRS complex), but on cessation of pacing a faster ventricular tachycardia with a different morphology has been induced.

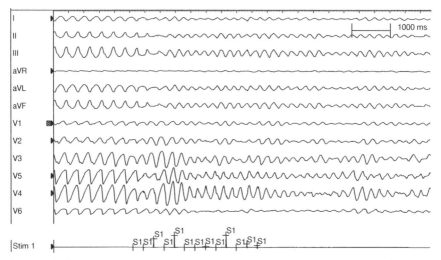

Figure 14.8 Continuation of the same patient as in Fig. 14.7. With ventricular pacing at a faster rate, the patient develops ventricular fibrillation and ultimately requires defibrillation (not shown).

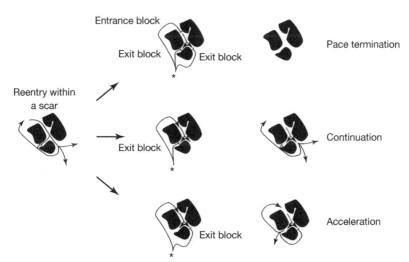

Figure 14.9 Schematic showing different responses to ventricular pacing, including no effect, acceleration, and termination.

Absence of structural heart disease

Electrocardiogram

The ECG is a fairly reliable tool for identifying the general region of a ventricular tachycardia focus in patients without structural heart disease. As a general rule, sites within the right ventricle will have a negative QRS complex in

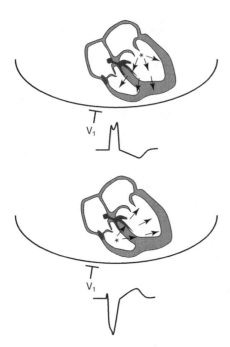

Figure 14.10 Ventricular tachycardias arising from the left ventricle will usually have a positive QRS complex in lead V_1, while ventricular tachycardias arising from the right ventricle will have a negative QRS complex.

lead V_1, because of the anterior location of the right ventricle within the chest (Fig. 14.10). Since the right ventricle is activated before the left ventricle, ventricular tachycardias arising from the right ventricle are often described as having a left bundle branch block morphology. In contrast, ventricular tachycardias arising from the left ventricle will have a predominantly positive QRS complex in V_1, because of the posterior location of the left ventricle. Since the left ventricle is activated before the right ventricle a broadly positive QRS complex in V_1 is often described as having a right bundle branch block morphology. Although there have been many case reports of ventricular tachycardias arising from almost all regions of both the left and right ventricles, most commonly they are found at one of three sites: the right ventricular outflow tract, the left ventricular outflow tract, and the midseptal region of the left ventricle (Table 14.1).

Right ventricular outflow tract

The right ventricular outflow tract is the most common site for idiopathic ventricular tachycardias (> 70%). The 12-lead ECG can be very helpful for identifying an arrhythmogenic focus within the right ventricular outflow tract and further localizing the exact arrhythmogenic site. The ECG in patients with a right ventricular outflow tract ventricular tachycardia will be characterized by a left bundle branch block morphology with broadly positive QRS complexes in the inferior leads (inferior axis) (Fig. 14.11).

Table 14.1 ECG characteristics of common idiopathic ventricular tachycardias.

Location	ECG characteristics
Right ventricular outflow tract	Left bundle branch block morphology in V_1
	Precordial transition in V_4
	Inferior axis
	Site from the free wall associated with a wider QRS complex
Left ventricular outflow tract	Right bundle branch block morphology in V_1
	Early precordial transition (V_2 at the latest)
	Inferior axis
	Septal sites with narrower QRS complexes, and may have left bundle branch block morphology in V_1
Left ventricular septum	Right bundle branch block morphology in V_1
	Superior axis

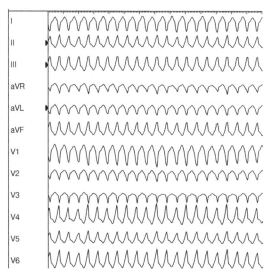

Figure 14.11 ECG from a patient with idiopathic ventricular tachycardia arising from the right ventricular outflow tract.

There are several ECG clues for further localizing the arrhythmogenic site within the outflow tract (Fig. 14.12). Sites on the anterior wall of the outflow tract will tend to have negative QRS complexes in both I and aVL, while posterior sites are more often characterized by a positive QRS in I and a negative QRS in aVL. Sites on the lateral wall will tend to have wider QRS complexes than septal sites because of later activation of the His–Purkinje tissue. For similar reasons, lower septal sites will tend to have less positive QRS complexes in

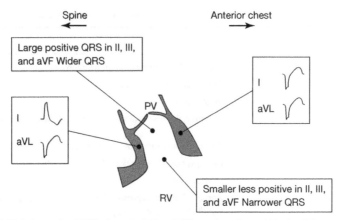

Figure 14.12 Schematic of ECG characteristics of different locations within the right ventricular outflow tract. In general, more superior sites that are farther from the normal His–Purkinje tissue will have wider more positive QRS complexes in the inferior leads. Posterior sites (closer to the spine) will tend to have a positive QRS complex in lead I. PV, pulmonary vein; RV, right ventricle.

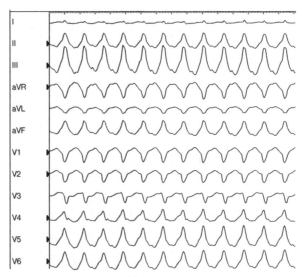

Figure 14.13 ECG from another patient with idiopathic ventricular tachycardia arising from the right ventricular outflow tract. This site was more posterior, yielding a positive QRS complex in lead I.

the inferior leads and narrower QRS complexes than sites higher in the outflow tract. Reexamine Fig. 14.10: this patient's focus was found to be in the anterior portion of the right ventricular outflow tract. The ECG in Fig. 14.13 is from another patient with right ventricular outflow tract tachycardia, although this site was located in the posterior portion of the outflow tract (notice the positive QRS complex in lead I).

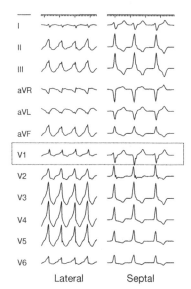

Figure 14.14 ECGs from two patients with left ventricular outflow tract sites. Left ventricular tachycardia will have a right bundle branch block morphology in V_1 (positive QRS complex) and an inferior axis. Sometimes tachycardias arising from the septal region will have a left bundle branch block morphology but an early precordial transition (point where the QRS becomes positive). In this case a positive QRS complex is noted in V_2. Also notice that the QRS complex is narrower in the septal site, presumably from partial activation of the His–Purkinje system.

Lateral   Septal

Left ventricular outflow tract

Tachycardias can also arise from the left ventricular outflow tract, although this is generally less frequently observed than the right ventricular outflow tract. Sites can be located below the aortic valve in the true left ventricular outflow tract, but at times are just above the aortic valve within the aortic cusps, presumably due to muscular extensions into the aorta and sinuses of Valsalva.

Ventricular tachycardia from a left ventricular outflow tract site will generally have a right bundle branch block pattern (positive QRS complex in V_1) with an inferior axis. Figure 14.14 shows 12-lead ECGs from two different patients with a left ventricular outflow tract ventricular tachycardia. In both ECGs the QRS axis is inferiorly directed, and positive concordance (left ECG) or early transition with a positive QRS complex in V_2 (right ECG) is noted in the precordial leads (see Chapter 6). In most cases, lead V_1 will have a right bundle branch morphology (positive QRS) in ventricular tachycardias from the left ventricular outflow tract. However, in some cases, sites from the septal portion of the left ventricular outflow tract will have a left bundle branch block pattern, but they will usually have an early transition, with positive R waves noted in V_2 (right ECG in Fig. 14.14).

Left ventricular septum

Ventricular tachycardias in normal hearts can also arise from the septal portion of the left ventricle. The ECG from a patient with septal ventricular tachycardia will have a right bundle branch block morphology (due to early activation of the left ventricle relative to the right), but will often have a superior axis. Figure 14.15 shows an example of a patient with a left septal ventricular tachycardia.

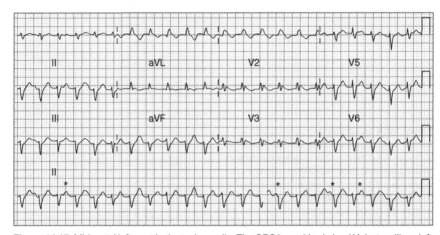

Figure 14.15 Midseptal left ventricular tachycardia. The QRS is positive in lead V_1 but, unlike a left ventricular outflow tract tachycardia, the QRS axis is superior.
(*) atrial activity dissociated from the QRS complexis can be seen.

Ablation

Ablation is effective for eliminating ventricular tachycardia in patients with structurally normal hearts, with success rates better than 70–80% depending on the site. In general, ablation of left ventricular sites can be more difficult than right ventricular sites (at least in part due to increased ventricular wall thickness), and it is associated with more significant complications (potential for cerebral embolus due to thrombus formation and increased risk of bleeding due to anticoagulation). Ablation within the right ventricular outflow tract can also be dangerous; death due to pericardial tamponade has been reported in the literature. However, despite these issues, radiofrequency catheter ablation is an effective treatment that should be considered as a potential first-line therapy in symptomatic patients with ventricular tachycardia or frequent premature ventricular contractions.

Ablation is performed by venous access for right ventricular sites, and using either a retrograde approach through the aorta or a transseptal approach for left ventricular sites. For a retrograde approach, the catheter is prolapsed through the aortic valve to reduce the risk of valve damage and to reduce the risk of the catheter tip engaging one of the coronary artery ostia. An example of an ablation catheter placed in the left ventricular outflow tract is shown in Fig. 14.16. Finally, in tertiary referral centers, epicardial ablation via catheters placed in the pericardial space is sometimes required for sites that cannot be reached with an endovascular approach.

Regardless of location, once the ablation catheter is in the area of interest, ablation is performed in the same manner. The easiest technique is to locate the earliest endocardial electrogram, usually preceding the onset of the earliest QRS by 15–45 ms. A patient with frequent symptomatic premature ventricular contractions arising from the right ventricular outflow tract is shown in Fig. 14.17. The ablation catheter is in a position with an early ventricular

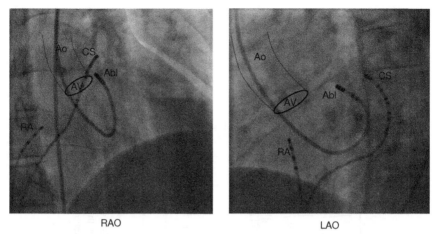

RAO   LAO

Figure 14.16 Right anterior oblique (RAO) and left anterior oblique (LAO) fluoroscopic images of ablation at the left ventricular outflow tract using a retrograde aortic approach. The approximate locations of the aortic valve (AV) and ascending aorta (Ao) are shown. Abl, ablation catheter; CS, coronary sinus catheter; RA, right atrial catheter.

electrogram and discrete potential that is associated with the premature ventricular contraction. Application of radiofrequency energy at this site results in prompt termination of the premature ventricular contractions. Oftentimes it is very useful to place specialized multielectrode catheters within the outflow tract to aid in identification of the earliest ventricular electrogram (Fig. 14.18). It is important to note that the potential may precede the QRS complex by a significant amount, particularly in patients with tachycardia sites in the left ventricular septum (Fig. 14.19).

Another technique that can be used in patients with structurally normal hearts is pacemapping. The basic concept is that pacing from the putative site of the tachycardia will yield a QRS complex that has exactly the same configuration as the QRS complex during ventricular tachycardia. Unfortunately, since the focus is surrounded by normal ventricular tissue with normal conduction properties, relatively large regions will have early electrograms and excellent pacemaps. Depending on the study, similar pacemaps can be obtained within areas as large as 2–3 cm^2. Despite this pitfall, pacemapping is an important technique for locating the catheter tip within the general "neighborhood," particularly in those patients with intermittent unsustained arrhythmias. An example of pacemapping in a patient with a right ventricular outflow tract tachycardia is shown in Fig. 14.20. The patient had only a single episode of sustained arrhythmia (left panel). Pacing was performed from the catheter tip in an attempt to identify the focus. Site #1 is too posterior and yields a positive QRS complex in lead I. Site #2, along the septum, improves the match in lead I but is too low in the septum with less positive narrower QRS complexes in leads II, III, and aVF and a later precordial transition (biphasic rather than a positive QRS in lead V$_4$). Moving the catheter to a more superior

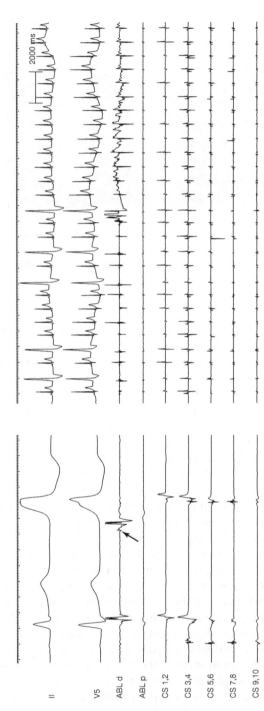

Figure 14.17 Mapping of the earliest endocardial signal for identifying a successful ablation site. In this patient with frequent premature ventricular contractions arising from the right ventricular outflow tract, a site with an early discrete signal associated with the premature ventricular contraction is identified (arrow). Application of radiofrequency energy results in prompt termination of the frequent premature ventricular contractions.

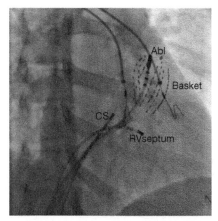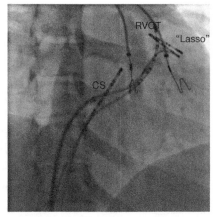

Figure 14.18 Use of complex multipolar catheters such as a circular "lasso" or basket catheter within the right ventricular outflow tract (RVOT) can facilitate endocardial mapping of ventricular tachycardias. Abl, ablation catheter; CS, coronary sinus catheter; RV septum, catheter at right ventricular septum.

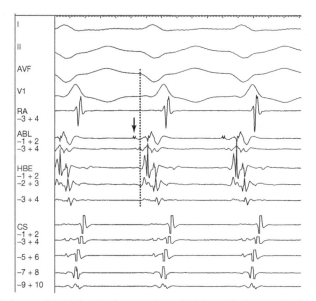

Figure 14.19 Successful ablation site from a patient with left ventricular septal tachycardia (right bundle branch block morphology, superior axis) was characterized by a discrete potential (arrow) that preceded the QRS by 22 ms.

site leads to site #3, which is an excellent match. Notice that not only does the general QRS morphology match (what's positive is positive, what's negative is negative), but all of the subtle deflections within the QRS complex are similar. After application of radiofrequency energy at this site the patient had no additional episodes of ventricular tachycardia even with extended follow-up.

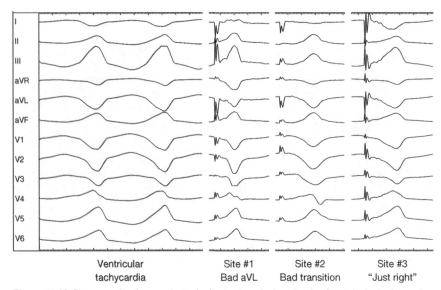

| Ventricular | Site #1 | Site #2 | Site #3 |
| tachycardia | Bad aVL | Bad transition | "Just right" |

Figure 14.20 Pacemapping for a patient who had only a single episode of ventricular tachycardia during the electrophysiology study. Pacemapping, by matching the QRS complex during pacing to the saved QRS complex during tachycardia, is one technique that can be used in this situation for identifying the tachycardia site.

Three-dimensional mapping systems have revolutionized ablation for ventricular tachycardia, because they allow the operator to target regions of interest and reliably return to those sites. In addition to mapping systems, ablation within the ventricle can also be facilitated by the use of large-tip catheters and irrigated-tip catheters, which allow larger lesions to be made (although with increased risk for perforation).

Presence of structural heart disease

Electrocardiogram

It is more difficult to use the ECG to localize sites of reentry for ventricular tachycardia in patients with structural heart disease, at least in part because of the great variability in substrates encountered in this condition. Since reentry is the most common mechanism for ventricular tachycardia in the setting of scar, the QRS morphology provides clues for the exit site for the reentrant circuit. Ventricular tachycardias with a left bundle branch block morphology will generally have an exit site in the septum, while a right bundle branch block morphology can be observed with ventricular tachycardias from any region within the left ventricle.

One unusual form of ventricular tachycardia that can be observed in patients with dilated cardiomyopathy is bundle branch reentry. In Chapter 3 we discussed how a single beat of bundle branch reentry can be observed.

In normal hearts, sustained bundle branch reentry is very rare, because rapid conduction through the bundles increases the likelihood that refractory ventricular tissue will be encountered, thus terminating the reentrant circuit. However, in patients with disease and slower conduction in the bundles, sustained bundle branch reentry can be observed. In the most common form of bundle branch reentry, the reentrant circuit involves retrograde conduction via the left bundle, anterograde conduction via the right bundle, and transseptal activation (Fig. 14.21). Figure 14.22 shows the ECG from a patient with bundle branch reentry. Since the ventricles are being activated solely by the right bundle a "pure left bundle branch block" pattern will be observed. Notice that atrioventricular dissociation is present, ruling out supraventricular tachycardia with aberrant conduction. In Fig. 14.23, the intracardiac electrograms

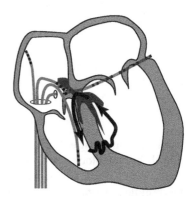

Figure 14.21 Schematic for bundle branch reentry. The most common form involves anterograde activation of the right bundle, transseptal right-to-left ventricular depolarization, and retrograde activation up the left bundle.

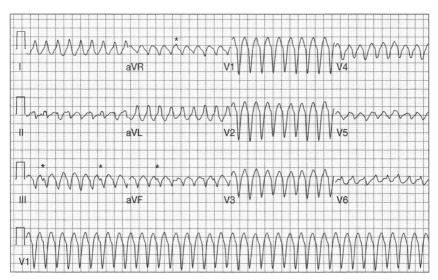

Figure 14.22 ECG from a patient with bundle branch reentry. A typical left bundle branch block morphology is observed. Atrioventricular dissociation can be observed, with "unexpected" deflections that must be due to atrial activity (*).

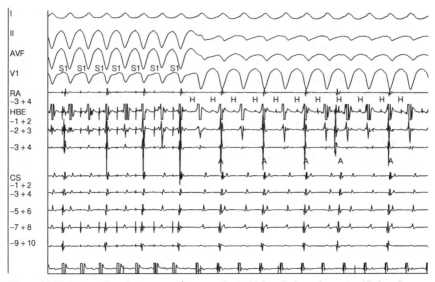

Figure 14.23 Intracardiac electrograms from a patient with bundle branch reentry. His bundle signals will be observed between QRS complexes, and changes in the HH interval will precede changes in the QRS interval.

from the same patient are shown. A wide complex tachycardia with a left bundle branch block morphology is initiated with ventricular pacing at a constant cycle length. Atrioventricular dissociation is present, but notice that a His bundle potential can be seen between the QRS complexes. The specific diagnosis of bundle branch reentry requires changes in the HH interval to precede changes in the interval between QRS complexes.

Electrophysiology and ablation

Ablation of ventricular tachycardia for patients with structural heart disease is approached differently than ablation in patients without structural heart disease. The main reason for this difference is the arrhythmia mechanism. In patients with structural heart disease, reentry is the most common reason for ventricular arrhythmias. Reentry is generally due to the presence of "channels" of viable tissue within scar. Ablation is focused on identifying critical channels during ventricular tachycardia (entrainment mapping) or during sinus rhythm (substrate mapping).

Preparation is extremely important in patients with structural heart disease undergoing ablation for ventricular tachycardia. Ventricular tachycardia in patients with structural heart disease can be associated with significant complications even in the best centers. In a large trial evaluating ablation of ventricular tachycardia, a significant complication rate of greater than 7% was reported, with a 3% risk of death within seven days of the procedure.

Identification of critical channels that may be contributing to the tachycardia can initially be based on the presence of diastolic activation. Figure 14.24

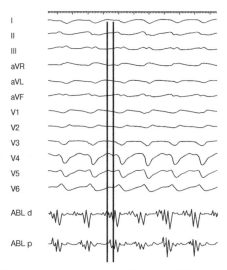

Figure 14.24 Intracardiac electrograms are recorded between QRS complexes (dotted lines) during ventricular tachycardia. Ablation at this site resulted in termination of the tachycardia.

shows electrograms from a site that is characterized by high-frequency signals during the period between QRS complexes (diastole). Ablation at this site resulted in termination of the tachycardia, but it should be noted that diastolic potentials can be observed at sites that are not involved in the reentrant circuit.

The critical isthmus of a reentrant circuit can be identified by the use of entrainment techniques, as described for atrial flutter in Chapter 12. Identification of entrainment is easier, because changes in QRS morphology are much easier to identify than changes in the P wave. If pacing is performed from a site away from the reentrant circuit, a change in the QRS complex will be observed, since the ventricles are being depolarized in a different pattern than during tachycardia. If pacing is performed within a critical isthmus the QRS complex during the paced beat will match the QRS complex during tachycardia (Figs. 14.25, 14.26). Sites near the exit site will have a short stimulus-to-QRS interval, while sites near the entrance site will have a longer stimulus-to-QRS interval. If pacing is occurring within the critical channel the interval between the stimulus and a fiduciary point (deflection of the QRS or a stable endocardial electrogram) will be the same as the interval between the recorded electrogram and the same fiduciary point. Figure 14.27 shows the intracardiac electrograms from this site. Ablation resulted in termination of the tachycardia after 12 seconds.

Substrate mapping

An important development over the past decade has been the realization that successful ablation could be accomplished by directly targeting the substrate for ventricular tachycardia. Using this technique, scar is usually classified as

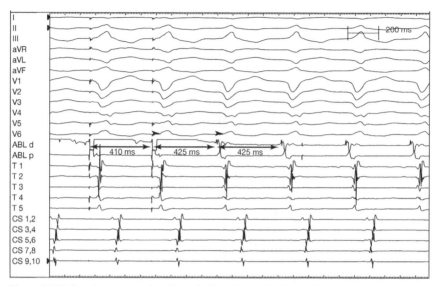

Figure 14.25 Entrainment mapping of ventricular tachycardia. Pacing during tachycardia yields almost the same QRS morphology as during tachycardia. The interval between the stimulus and an endocardial signal recorded from a distant site matches the interval between the electrogram and the endocardial signal (arrowheads). In addition, the interval between the last paced beat and the first electrogram will be the same as the tachycardia cycle length (double-headed arrows).

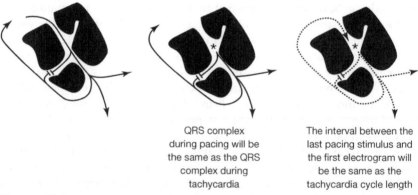

QRS complex during pacing will be the same as the QRS complex during tachycardia

The interval between the last pacing stimulus and the first electrogram will be the same as the tachycardia cycle length

Figure 14.26 If pacing is performed within the critical isthmus used for reentry, pacing will yield a QRS complex that is the same as the tachycardia QRS, and the interval between the last paced beat and the first electrogram will be the same as the tachycardia interval, since the path of depolarization in both cases is the same (dashed line).

regions with attenuated electrograms (< 1.5 mV), with dense scar identified by an even lower electrogram amplitude (< 0.5 mV) and inability to pace despite high outputs (> 10 mA). Ablation is performed at viable tissue within scars or by creating linear lesions between scars. Three-dimensional mapping techniques have made this ablation technique feasible, because individual sites

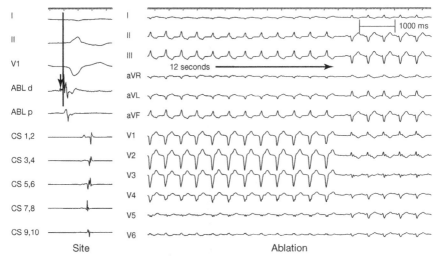

Figure 14.27 Electrograms from the same site as Fig. 14.25. The endocardial electrogram (arrow) precedes the upstroke of the QRS complex. Radiofrequency energy resulted in termination of the tachycardia after 12 seconds.

Figure 14.28 Pacing from a ventricular site adjacent to the mitral valve yields a QRS morphology that matches the ventricular tachycardia, suggesting similar exit sites. The interval from stimulus to a fiduciary point (in this case an endocardial ventricular electrogram is used) is the same as the interval from electrogram to fiduciary point. The short interval between the stimulus/endocardial electrogram and the initial upstroke of the QRS complex suggests that the ablation catheter is within the critical isthmus near the exit site. A pacing artifact that does not lead to capture can be seen in the second QRS complex.

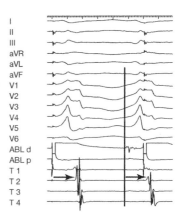

can be stored and integrated with information from adjacent cardiac tissue to accurately delineate scars and return to areas of interest.

Oftentimes a combination of techniques is required for a single patient. Figure 14.28 shows the electrogram and QRS complex from a left ventricular region adjacent to the mitral valve during pacing and ventricular tachycardia. In the patient presented in Fig. 14.28, it appeared that a critical isthmus between scar from a prior myocardial infarction and the mitral valve was present during ventricular tachycardia. Unfortunately the patient continually deteriorated to ventricular fibrillation or rapid ventricular tachycardia requiring external shocks (Fig. 14.29). For this reason substrate mapping was

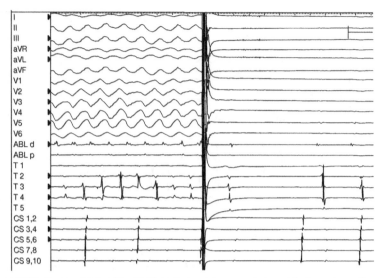

Figure 14.29 Same patient as Fig. 14.28. Unfortunately, every time ventricular tachycardia was induced the patient would quickly deteriorate to ventricular fibrillation requiring defibrillation.

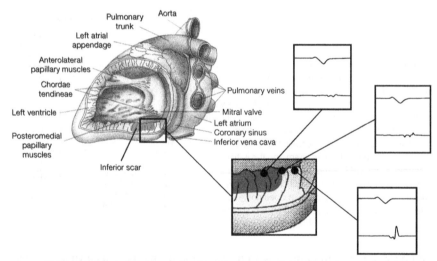

Figure 14.30 Mapping during sinus rhythm identified an area of dense scar from a prior inferior wall myocardial infarction. The electrograms were low-amplitude and could not be paced despite high outputs (10 mA). During sinus rhythm, a linear ablation was performed connecting the inferior scar to the mitral valve. After ablation the patient was not inducible for ventricular arrhythmias. (Adapted from Kusumoto FM. Cardiovascular disorders: heart disease. In: McPhee SJ, Lingappa VR, Ganong WF, eds. *Pathophysiology of Disease*, 5th edn. New York, NY: McGraw-Hill, 2003.)

performed, with scar identified by delineating regions with attenuated electrograms. Ablation was performed during sinus rhythm between the scar and the mitral valve (Fig. 14.30). After ablation the patient was noninducible and has not had subsequent arrhythmias.

CHAPTER 15

Implantable cardiac devices: ECGs and electrograms

Implantable cardiac devices for the management of arrhythmias have become a standard therapy for a variety of clinical conditions. Although a comprehensive discussion of device therapy is far beyond the scope of this book, since devices use leads that are essentially "permanent electrophysiology catheters," evaluation of electrograms obtained from devices and ECG changes associated with pacing are cogent to our discussion.

Pacing

Intrinsic cardiac activity produced by the heart (electrograms) are recorded, analyzed, and stored by cardiac devices. Most devices allow both bipolar electrograms (recorded from two electrodes within the chamber where the lead is located) and unipolar electrograms (recorded from a tip electrode located within the heart and the device "can" itself, located in the upper shoulder). Figure 15.1 shows examples of bipolar and unipolar electrograms recorded from a lead placed in the atrium and a lead placed in the ventricle. Since the unipolar leads record over a larger distance, far-field ventricular activity is recorded in the atrial lead and T waves are more prominent in the ventricular lead.

Atrial pacing
Pacing from atrial leads will produce P waves (Fig. 15.2). Since atrial leads are normally placed within the right atrial appendage near the sinus node, the P waves are usually upright and are similar in shape to the P waves observed during sinus rhythm. However, pacing leads can be placed in any position. The resultant P wave from a lead placed in the low lateral wall of the right atrium is also shown in Fig. 15.2. Notice that the P wave is no longer upright in the inferior leads.

Right ventricular pacing
Pacing from ventricular leads will produce QRS complexes. Pacing leads have traditionally been placed in the inferior portion of the right ventricular apex,

Understanding Intracardiac EGMs and ECGs. By Fred Kusumoto. Published 2010 by Blackwell Publishing. ISBN: 978-1-4051-8410-6

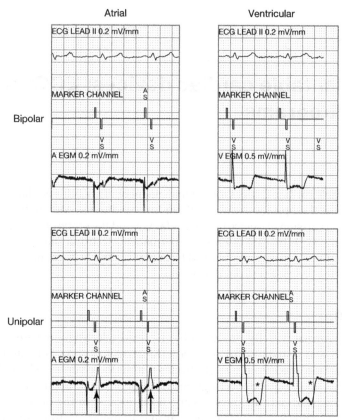

Figure 15.1 Electrograms recorded from an atrial pacing lead and a ventricular pacing lead in bipolar and unipolar modes. In the atrial electrogram, far-field ventricular activity (arrows) can be observed in the unipolar mode. In the ventricular lead, the ventricular electrogram is wider, and more prominent signals due to ventricular repolarization (*) are observed.

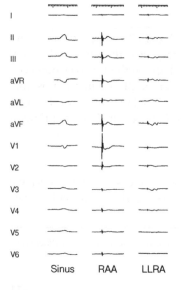

Figure 15.2 P waves from the same patient during sinus rhythm, and during pacing from the right atrial appendage (RAA) and the low lateral right atrium (LLRA).

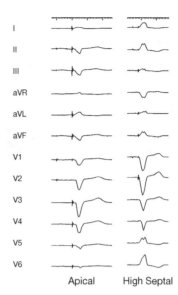

Figure 15.3 Effects of different pacing sites in the right ventricle on the QRS complex. Pacing from the inferior apex usually produces a left bundle branch block pattern with negative concordance or a late transition and a superior axis (negative QRS complexes in the inferior leads). Pacing from higher in the septal region still produces a left bundle branch block morphology but a more normal transition and a normal or rightward axis.

which leads to a paced QRS complex that has a left bundle branch block morphology with negative concordance or a late transition in the precordial leads and a superior axis (Fig. 15.3). With the realization that pacing from the right ventricular apex can produce deleterious hemodynamic effects in some patients, many implanting physicians place ventricular leads in the mid septum or high septum. Pacing from the mid septum or high septum of the right ventricle still produces a QRS with a left bundle branch block morphology in V_1, but usually with a more normal precordial transition and a normal or slightly rightward axis (Fig. 15.3).

Fluoroscopy is important for permanent lead placement. Figure 15.4 shows fluoroscopic positions of right ventricular leads placed at the midseptal region and the inferior apex. A coronary sinus venogram shows the position of the coronary sinus os and the left-sided chambers. In the first two panels fluoroscopic images of a defibrillator lead in the midseptum and a pacing lead in the right ventricular apex are shown in the left anterior oblique (LAO) and right anterior oblique (RAO) orientations. In the third panel, an LAO image of a lead that has been inadvertently placed in the left ventricle is shown. In this panel, a temporary pacing lead can be seen in the right ventricle. These images emphasize the importance of evaluating fluoroscopic images in the left anterior oblique position to confirm appropriate placement of pacing leads.

Sometimes permanent pacing leads will become partially or completely dislodged, or associated with poor pacing function due to the development of scar tissue around the lead. An example of intermittent capture of a right ventricular lead is shown in Fig. 15.5. The ventricular lead is placed relatively high in the right ventricular septum (QRS with a left bundle branch block morphology and an inferior axis). Intermittently the ventricular pacing stimulus

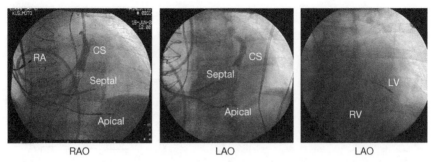

Figure 15.4 Fluoroscopic images of different ventricular lead positions. The first two panels show right anterior oblique (RAO) and left anterior oblique (LAO) images of correctly positioned leads in the septal portion of the right ventricular apex and septum. Angiography of the coronary sinus (CS) shows the position of the coronary sinus os and outlines left-sided structures (remember that the coronary sinus travels in the groove separating the left atrium from the left ventricle. The third panel shows an LAO image of a lead that has been inadvertently placed in the left ventricle (LV), with a temporary pacing lead in the right ventricle (RV).

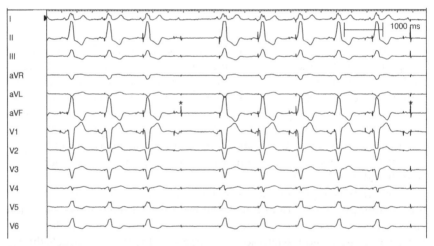

Figure 15.5 ECG showing intermittent ventricular capture. Intermittently a pacing stimulus does not lead to ventricular depolarization (failure to capture) and no QRS is produced (*).

does not lead to ventricular capture and a QRS complex is not observed. Although the pacing output can be increased, in many cases the lead position must be revised.

Biventricular pacing

Pacing has now developed into an adjunctive treatment for patients with heart failure and cardiac dyssynchrony. Some patients with reduced left ventricular function will also have significant delays in ventricular activation of the lateral wall of the left ventricle. Dyssynchronous ventricular contraction can

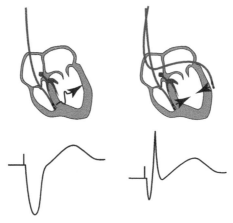

Figure 15.6 Schematic showing the potential advantage of biventricular pacing over pacing from the right ventricle.

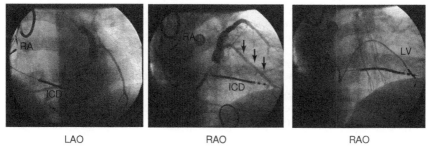

LAO   RAO   RAO

Figure 15.7 Fluoroscopy in the left anterior oblique (LAO) and right anterior oblique (RAO) of the coronary sinus and its branches. A large branch on the lateral wall is chosen for lead placement (arrows), and the third panel shows a ventricular lead placed in this venous branch.

be associated with inefficient cardiac function. Biventricular pacing – pacing simultaneously from the right ventricle and the left ventricle – can help "resynchronize" ventricular contraction (Fig. 15.6).

Biventricular pacing is performed by placing a lead in a branch of the coronary sinus (Fig. 15.7). Usually placement of the left ventricular lead is performed by injecting contrast into the coronary sinus and identifying target veins on the lateral wall. Pacing leads are placed in the desired branch using a series of sheaths, catheters, and guidewires (and sometimes good luck).

The effects of biventricular pacing on the surface ECG are illustrated in Fig. 15.8, showing a patient who has a very wide QRS complex (215 ms) with a left bundle branch block morphology at baseline. In a patient with heart failure and reduced left ventricular function, the wide QRS suggests that depolarization of the left ventricle takes a significant amount of time and that

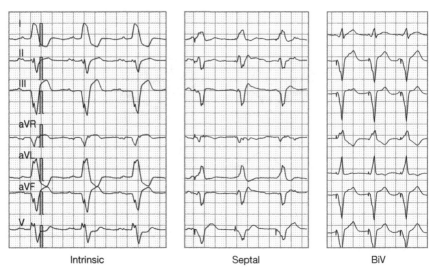

| Intrinsic | Septal | BiV |

Figure 15.8 Effects of pacing on QRS morphology. At baseline the patient has a very wide QRS complex with a left bundle branch block morphology. Septal pacing from the right ventricle decreases the QRS complex slightly, but biventricular pacing (BiV) is associated with a significant decrease in the QRS width, suggesting more coordinated ventricular contraction.

cardiac dyssynchrony is present. With septal pacing, the QRS interval is slightly decreased, but with biventricular pacing a significant decrease in the QRS width is observed, suggesting more coordinated and simultaneous depolarization of the ventricles.

Monitoring and treatment of tachyarrhythmias

Modern implantable devices have extensive memory and multiple functions and features that the clinician can use to optimize treatment for an individual patient. One of the important features of devices is the ability to record and store episodes of arrhythmia. Figure 15.9 shows electrograms from stored events in two different patients complaining of episodes of rapid heart rates. In the top panel, the rapid heart rate is initiated with a premature atrial contraction, and the ventricular electrograms during tachycardia are similar to the ventricular electrograms during sinus rhythm. Both of these findings suggest that a nonsustained atrial tachycardia was present. In contrast, in the bottom panel, the episode of tachycardia is initiated with a premature ventricular contraction. The presence of atrioventricular dissociation confirms the diagnosis of nonsustained ventricular tachycardia.

If arrhythmias are sustained, defibrillators and some pacemakers are designed to automatically detect and terminate arrhythmias. Figure 15.10 shows a stored electrogram from a patient with prior myocardial infarction and reduced left ventricular function. In this case the defibrillator detects the rapid

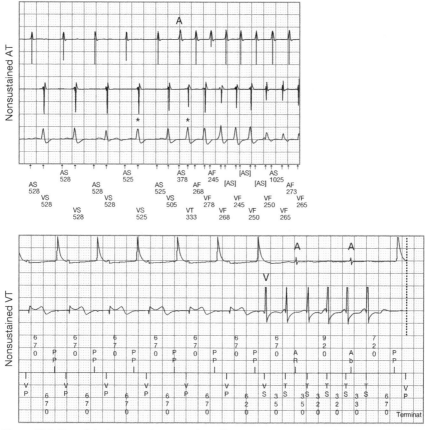

Figure 15.9 Stored electrograms that are retrieved from the implanted device's memory. *Top:* Electrograms suggest an episode of atrial fibrillation. The tachycardia is initiated with a premature atrial complex (A), and the ventricular electrograms (*) are the same during both tachycardia and sinus rhythm, suggesting a similar depolarization sequence in both conditions. *Bottom:* The tachycardia is initiated by a premature ventricular contraction (V), and the presence of atrioventricular dissociation confirms the presence of nonsustained ventricular tachycardia.

abnormal heart rate and delivers a burst of ventricular pacing that terminates the tachycardia.

Some devices also have a manual function that essentially allows the clinician to perform a rudimentary electrophysiology procedure using the device leads. Figure 15.11 shows the 12-lead ECG of a patient with sustained supraventricular tachycardia. Although suggested by the ECG, the atrial electrograms obtained from the device confirm the presence of atrial activity just after the QRS (Fig. 15.12). The short VA conduction time rules out an accessory pathway-mediated tachycardia. Termination of the tachycardia with ventricular pacing (Fig. 15.13) suggests that the patient had supraventricular tachycardia due to AV node reentry.

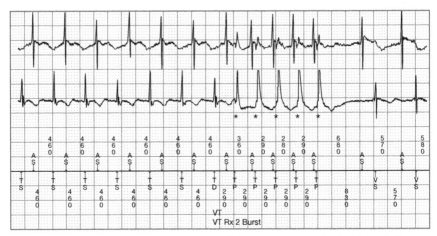

Figure 15.10 Automatic detection and treatment of ventricular tachycardia. Rapid ventricular activity is identified by the device (TS, tachycardia sense), and once a critical number is reached the device "detects" tachycardia (TD, tachycardia detect). The device has been programmed to deliver a short burst of ventricular pacing (*) (TP, tachycardia pace) that results in termination of the ventricular tachycardia. Notice that the ventricular electrogram during tachycardia is different from the ventricular electrogram in sinus rhythm because of different depolarization direction.

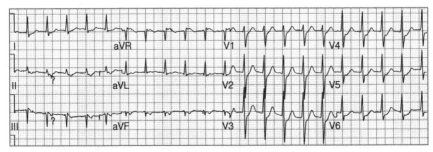

Figure 15.11 ECG from a patient with supraventricular tachycardia. A terminal deflection in the QRS complex (?) may represent atrial activity.

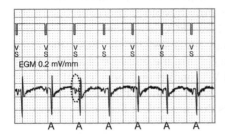

Figure 15.12 Atrial electrograms during tachycardia confirm the presence of atrial activity (A) immediately after ventricular sensed activity (VS, ventricular sense). Far-field signal due to ventricular activity can be seen (circled).

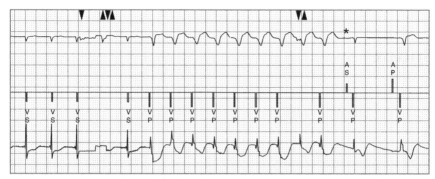

Figure 15.13 Ventricular pacing performed manually by the clinician terminates the tachycardia (VS, ventricular sense) and returns the patient to sinus rhythm with a P wave (*) preceding ventricular pacing (VP).

Index

Page numbers in **bold** represent tables, those in *italics* represent figures.

ablation 99–103
  accessory pathways 125–9, *126–9*
  atrial flutter *162, 170, 172*
    eustachian ridge *171*
    pouch *171*
  AV node reentry 142–7, *143–6*
  cryothermal 103
  focal atrial tachycardia 154–60, *155–9*
  radiofrequency 99–101, *100–2*
    irrigated 101–3, *102, 103*
  supraventricular tachycardia *128*
  ventricular pacing *127*
  ventricular tachycardia 200–4, *201–4*
    structural heart disease 206–7, *207*
accessory pathways 107–31
  ablation 125–9, *126–9*
  anatomy 107–8, **108**
  ECG 108–14
    sinus rhythm 108–12, *109–12*
    tachycardia 112–14, *112–14*
  electrophysiology 107–8, **108**, 114–25
    atrial pacing 115–20, *115–19*
    baseline evaluation 114
    tachycardia 122–5, *123–5*
    ventricular pacing 120–2, *121, 122*
  slow conducting 130–1, *131*
  types of **108**
  unusual 129–31, *129–31*
adenosine 148
  response to 82, *82*
AH interval 25, *25*
anterior-posterior orientation *20*
antidromic AV reentrant tachycardia 112, *113*
arrhythmias
  evaluation of **50**
  see also *individual arrhythmias*

atrial activation 70–4, *72, 73*
  eccentric 71
  temporal relationships 74
atrial delayed conduction **36**
atrial eccentric depolarization 121
atrial effective refractory period *38*, **39**, *40*
atrial extrastimulus 36, **36, 50**
atrial fibrillation 62, 65, 113, 182–8
  ECG *90, 154*, 182–3, *183*
  electrogram *70*
  electrophysiology 183–8, *183–8*
  mechanism 182
atrial flutter 62, 66, 148, 161–81
  ablation *162, 170, 172*
    eustachian ridge *171*
    pouch *171*
  cavotricuspid isthmus-dependent 163–73, *164–73*
  cavotricuspid isthmus-independent 174–81, *174–81*
  clockwise 169, *170*
  ECG *73, 150, 165*
  evaluation and treatment **162**
  mechanism 161–3, *162*, **162**
  see also focal atrial tachycardia
atrial pacing **50**, 211, *212*
  accessory pathways 115–20, *115–19*
  AV node reentry 134–7, *135–7*
  overdrive 30, 32–4, *32–4*
atrial premature beats 80–2, *81, 82*
atrial premature stimulation 34–42, *35–42*, **36**
atrial tachycardia *80*, **85**
  focal 62
  multifocal 62
  P wave in *67*
  with rapid anterograde conduction *112*
atrioventricular see AV

atrium *see* left atrium; right atrium
automaticity 60–2
    triggered activity 62
AV block *34*
AV conduction block 52–9
    baseline evaluation 52–5, *53–6*
    cycle length 55–7, *56*, *57*
    refractoriness 56–9, *57–9*
AV dissociation 88, *88*, *89*
AV node 25, *25*
    anatomy *133*
    delayed conduction **36**
    retrograde conduction *45*
AV node reentry 62, 64, *80*, **85**, 132–47
    ablation 142–7, *143–6*
    anatomy and electrophysiology 132–3,
        133
    atypical 141–2, *142*
    ECG 133–4, *134*
    electrophysiology 134–42
        atrial pacing 134–7, *135–7*
        tachycardia 139–42, *140–2*
        ventricular pacing 137–9, *138*, *139*
    orthodromic 64
    P wave in *67*
AV reentrant tachycardia 139–42, *140–2*
    antidromic 112, 113, *113*, *114*
    orthodromic 112, *113*, *123*
AV reentry *80*
    accessory pathways **85**
AV refractory period *38*, **39**, *40*

Bachmann's bundle 149
baseline recording **50**
bipolar recording 11–12, *12*
biventricular pacing 214–16, *215*, *216*
brady-tachy syndrome 51
bradycardia 51–9
    AV conduction block 52–9
    sinus node dysfunction 51–2, *52*
Brockenbrough needle 6, *7*
bundle branch block *124*
    ECG *87*
bundle branch reentry *46*, *205*, *206*

catheter location/mapping systems
        95–8
    magnetic positioning 95–6, *96*
    noncontact mapping 96–8, *97*

catheters 10–11, *11*
    Cournand *11*
    Josephson *11*
    positioning *15*
cavotricuspid isthmus-dependent atrial
        flutter 163–73, *164–73*
cavotricuspid isthmus-independent atrial
        flutter 174–81, *174–81*
chamber access 5–10, *5–10*
complex fractionated atrial electrograms
        184–5, *186*
coronary sinus 5, *5*, 16, *17*, *18*
    os 149, **150**
Coumel's sign 125
Cournand catheter *11*
crista terminalis 148, **150**
critical isthmus 161, 174
cryothermal ablation 103

decremental conduction 33
delayed conduction
    atrial *36*
    AV node **36**
    His-Purkinje system **36**
delta waves *see* sinus rhythm

eccentric activation 71, 121
ECG
    accessory pathways 108–14
    atrial fibrillation *90*, *154*, 182–3, *183*
    atrial flutter *73*, *150*, *165*
    AV node reentry 133–4, *134*
    bundle branch block *87*
    electrophysiologic evaluation 89–93
    focal atrial tachycardia 149–51,
        149–51, **150**
    normal 22–8, *23–7*
    supraventricular tachycardia 64–8, *81*
    ventricular tachycardia *88*, 195–200,
        197
        left ventricular outflow tract 199, *199*
        left ventricular septum 199, *200*
        right ventricular outflow tract
            196–9, *197–9*
        structural heart disease 204–6, *205*,
            206
    wide complex tachycardia 86–9, *87–9*
echocardiography 94–5, *95*
electrocardiogram *see* ECG

electrogram 23, 24
  atrial fibrillation 70
  atrial flutter 73
  His signal 27
  right bundle potential 27
  supraventricular tachycardia 69–74,
    70, 72, 81
    atrial activation 70–4, 72, 73
    evaluation **84**
    temporal relationships 74
  see also electrophysiology
electrophysiology 22–8, 23–7
  accessory pathways 114–25
    atrial pacing 115–20, 115–19
    baseline evaluation 114
    tachycardia 122–5, 123–5
    ventricular pacing 120–2, 121, 122
  atrial fibrillation 183–8, 183–8
  AV node reentry 134–42
  components of **50**
  focal atrial tachycardia 148–9, 151–4,
    152, 153
  signal acquisition 11–14, 12–14
  supraventricular tachycardia 68–82,
    85
    during tachycardia 69–74
    initiation and spontaneous
      termination 75–6
    response to drugs 82
    response to stimuli 76–82
entrainment mapping 164, 206

fasciculoventricular fibers 129–30, 129,
    130
femoral artery 3
femoral vein cannulation 3
filters 13–14, 13, 14
fluoroscopic anatomy 15–22, 16–22
  left anterior oblique view 17, 19, 20, 21,
    22
  right anterior oblique view 17, 19, 20, 21
focal atrial tachycardia 62, 148–60
  anatomy 148–9
  ECG 149–51, 149–51, **150**
  electrophysiology 148–9, 151–4, 152,
    153
  mapping and ablation 154–60, 155–9

gap phenomenon 57

heart
  anatomy 5
  chambers 15
high-pass filters 13
His bundle 18, 18
  effective refractory period 56, 57
  signal electrogram 27
His-Purkinje system, delayed conduction
    36
HV interval 25, 25, 52
  prolonged 55

implantable cardiac devices 211–19
  pacing see pacing
  tachycardias 216–19, 217–19
infraHisian block 54, 55, 56, 58, 59
infraHisian refractoriness 38
inguinal crease 3
inguinal ligament 3
intraHisian delay 57, 57

Josephson catheter 11
junctional ectopic tachycardia 62

Koch's triangle 149

left anterior oblique orientation 17, 19,
    20, 21, 22, 22
left atrial access 5–9, 5–10
left atrium 17
  vascular access 6–10, 7–10
left ventricle 17
left ventricular access 9–10
left ventricular outflow tract tachycardia
    199, 199
left ventricular septal tachycardia 199, 200
low-pass filters 13

magnetic positioning of catheters 95–6,
    96, 97
mapping
  accessory pathways 125
  anterograde 125, 126
  catheter systems 95–8
  entrainment 164, 206
  focal atrial tachycardia 154–60, 155–9
  retrograde 125
  ventricular pacing 127
  ventricular tachycardia 207–10, 208–10

mapping (*continued*)
  see also catheter location/mapping
    systems
microreentry 163
mitral annulus **150**
Mullins sheath/introducer 6, 6
multifocal atrial tachycardia 62

narrow complex tachycardia *112*
normal ECG 22–8, *23–7*
notch filters 13

orthodromic AV reentrant tachycardia
  112, *112*, *113*, *123*

P wave 66
  atrial tachycardia *67*, *68*, *68*
  AV reentry *67*
  sinus rhythm *67*
pacemaker cells 61
pacing **29**, 30–47, *31*, 211–16, *212*
  atrial **50**, 211, *212*
    overdrive 30, 32–4, *32–4*
  atrial premature stimulation 34–42,
    34–42
  biventricular 214–16, *215*, *216*
  tachycardia 47–9, *47–9*
  ventricular **50**
    right 211, 213–14, *213*, *214*
  ventricular overdrive 42–4, *43*
  ventricular premature stimulation
    44–7, *45*, *46*
patent foramen ovale 8
PR interval 26
  prolonged *53*, *54*
premature beats 27–8, *27*
programmed stimulation 29–50
  baseline pacing **29**, 30–47, *31*
  pacing during tachycardia 47–9, *47–9*
pulmonary veins **150**, *185*
Purkinje fibres *25*, *26*

QRS complex 26, *26*, 28
  accessory pathways 108–10, *109–11*
  atrial tachycardia 66
  widening of **36**

radiofrequency ablation 99–101, *100–2*
  irrigated 101–3, *102*, *103*

reentry 62
refractoriness 34, *35*
refractory period 35
  absolute 35
  calculation of **39**
  characteristics **39**
  effective 36–7, *38*
  relative 36
right anterior oblique orientation 17, *19*,
  20, *21*, 22
right atrium *16*
  activation 24
  high 18
right bundle potential 27
right ventricle *16*
right ventricular outflow tract
  tachycardia 196–9, *197–9*
right ventricular pacing 211, 213–14, *213*,
  214
robotic navigation 98

saphenous vein 3
sensing 47
signal acquisition 11–14, *12–14*
sinus node 24
  dysfunction 51–2, *52*
  recovery time 51, *52*
sinus rhythm 108–12, *109–12*
  P wave *67*
sinus tachycardia 61
superficial femoral artery 3
supraventricular tachycardia 60–85
  ablation 128
  anatomic classification 62–4, *63*
  atrial premature beats 80–2, *81*, *82*
  AV node reentry 135
  cellular and tissue classification 60–2,
    61
  differential diagnosis **85**
  ECG 64–8, *81*
  electrogram 69–74, *70*, *72*, *81*
    atrial activation 70–4, *72*, *73*
    evaluation **84**
    temporal relationships 74
  electrophysiology 68–83, *85*
  initiation and spontaneous termination
    75–6, *75*, *76*
  irregular 64–5, *65*
  regular 65–8, *65–9*

supraventricular tachycardia (*continued*)
  response to drugs 82, *83*
  ventricular premature beats 76–80,
      77–80
syncope *59*

T wave *66*
tachycardia
  accessory pathways
    ECG 112–14, *112–14*
    electrophysiology 122–5, *123–5*
  AV reentrant 139–42, *140–2*
    antidromic 112, 113, *113, 114*
    orthodromic 112, *113, 123*
  evaluation **29**
  focal atrial 148–60
  implantable cardiac devices 216–19,
      217–19
  junctional ectopic *62*
  narrow complex *112*
  orthodromic AV reentrant *112*
  pacing 47–9, *47–9*
  supraventricular *see* supraventricular
      tachycardia
  ventricular *see* ventricular tachycardia
  wide complex 86–93, *112*
Todaro's tendon *133*
triangle of Koch 132, *133*
tricuspid annulus 149
triggered activity *62*

unipolar recording 11–12, *12*

vascular access 3–5, *4*
ventricular activation, temporal
    relationships 74
ventricular depolarization *26*
ventricular effective refractory period **39**,
    191

ventricular extrastimuli **50**
ventricular fibrillation *192, 195*
ventricular overdrive pacing 42–4, *43*
ventricular pacing **50**, *194, 195*
  ablation *127*
  accessory pathways 120–2, *121, 122*
  AV node reentry 137–9, *138, 139*
  biventricular 214–16, *215, 216*
  mapping during *127*
  responses to *195*
  right ventricle 211, 213–14, *213, 214*
ventricular premature beats 76–80,
    77–80
ventricular premature stimulation 44–7,
    45, 46
ventricular tachycardia *91*, 189–210
  ablation 200–4, *201–4*
    structural heart disease 206–7, *207*
  AV dissociation *88*
  ECG *88*, 195–200, **197**
    left ventricular outflow tract 199, *199*
    left ventricular septum 199, *200*
    right ventricular outflow tract
        196–9, *197–9*
    structural heart disease 204–6, *205,
        206*
  electrophysiology 206–7, *207*
  mechanism 189–95, *190–5*
  substrate mapping 207–10, *208–10*
ventriculoatrial effective refractory
    period **39**, *45*

Wenckebach block 33, 34, *34*
wide complex tachycardia 86–93, *112*
  atrial vs ventricular activity 89–91, *90,
      91*
  causes *87*
  ECG 86–9, *87–9*
  initiation and termination 91–3, *92*

Printed and bound by CPI Group (UK) Ltd, Croydon, CR0 4YY

27/10/2024

14580191-0001